# The Extracellular Matrix and Cancer

## Regulation of Tumor Cell Biology by Tenascin-C

**Edited by**

**Gertraud Orend**
*Institut National de la Santé et de la Recherche Médicale, France*

**Falk Saupe**
*Institut National de la Santé et de la Recherche Médicale, France*

**Anja Schwenzer**
*Institut National de la Santé et de la Recherche Médicale, France*

**Kim Midwood**
*Oxford University, United Kingdom*

The Extracellular Matrix and Cancer – Regulation of Tumor Cell Biology by Tenascin-C

Publisher: iConcept Press Ltd.
Cover design: Pineapple Design Ltd.
Interior design: iConcept Press Ltd.
Typesetting and copy editing: iConcept Press Ltd. and Pineapple Design Ltd.

ISBN: 978-1-922227-522

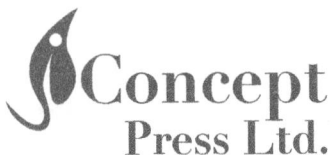

$\mathcal{J}$Concept
Press Ltd.

www.iconceptpress.com

# Preface

*"When a plant goes to seed, its seeds are*
*carried in all directions; but they can only live*
*and grow if they fall on congenial soil"*
*- Stephen Paget, 1889*

Cancer remains one of the biggest threats to our ever-increasing population; few lives remain untouched by this disease. An estimated 12.7 million new cases were diagnosed worldwide in 2008 and cancer caused an estimated 7.6 million deaths in the same year (IACR, 2008; WHO, 2008). Most of these deaths are a result of cancer that has spread from the original lesion to colonize a new site in the body; indeed metastatic cancers remain the most difficult to treat, with the worst prognoses.

Prompted by the observation that different cancers actually spread to very specific and often very distinct secondary sites, Paget first proposed his 'seed and soil' hypothesis to explain this phenomenon over a century ago. His paper highlighted for the first time the importance of the environment or 'the soil' in supporting the dissemination of cancer cells, 'the seed'. Since then an army of researchers around the globe have begun to investigate in greater mechanistic detail precisely how the environment of, not only the metastatic cancer cell, but also the primary cancer cell, dictates disease pathogenesis. Their discoveries have shed light on how the extracellular matrix surrounding and supporting cancer cells is key to driving cancer progression.

Here we focus on the progress in our understanding of how one component of the tumor soil, tenascin-C, is responsible for promoting the survival of primary tumor cells. We also review data that reveal a new role for tenascin-C in promoting tumor angiogenesis and enabling the migrating metastatic cancer cell to thrive at secondary tumor sites. Finally, we highlight how this work has opened the door for a variety of new therapeutic interventions that may help to treat cancer.

## Acknowledgements

We would like to acknowledge Christane Arnold for technical assistance, Dominique Guenot and the Hôpital Hautepierre for providing human colorectal carcinoma tissue. FS was supported by the Fondation des Treilles. AS was supported by a grant from the University Strasbourg and the Association pour la recherche sur le cancer (ARC). GO is supported by grants from INSERM, University Strasbourg, Ligue contre le Cancer, ANR and INCa. KM is supported by Arthritis Research UK.

# Contents

# Contents

# Chapter 1

# Background

The environment within which cancer cells exist is a key determinant of tumor survival and growth. The extracellular matrix that comprises the tumor stroma provides vital cues that control cell phenotype and enable the tumor to thrive. Moreover, emerging evidence reveals the importance of the extracellular matrix in permitting colonization of secondary tumor sites by creating a specific environmental niche tailored to enhance metastatic cell survival. Tenascin-C is an extracellular matrix glycoprotein whose expression is specifically induced in many different types of cancer where it drives processes such as tumor cell growth, angiogenesis, immune modulation and metastatic fitness. Here, we review the molecular mechanisms underlying the pleiotrophic role of tenascin-C in disease pathology and highlight the impact of these data on the development of new strategies to diagnose and treat cancer.

The extracellular matrix is a complex three-dimensional (3D) network of secreted molecules that provides structural support to tissues and which dynamically and reciprocally communicates with cells in order to regulate cell behaviour. Established during embryonic development to guide morphogenesis and maintained in adults to define tissue architecture and to support tissue homeostasis, it has long been established that the extracellular matrix undergoes profound changes during tumorigenesis. More recently, the idea that the expression, or re-expression, of specific matrix molecules in cancer forms a tumorigenic niche creating an environment that supports tumor growth has emerged. This environment impacts the phenotype of both tumor cells and stromal cells enabling survival and expansion of the primary tumor, as well as mediating the escape of metastatic tumor cells and their colonization of new sites at distinct and specific tissue locations. The extracellular matrix does this by virtue of a number of functions; it serves to anchor cells, it can provide either a migration barrier or a migration track to control cell movement, it directly interacts with the cell to provide external cues, it acts as a reservoir for soluble signaling molecules controlling their localization and concentration, often additionally serving as a co-receptor or presenter of these molecules at the cell surface, and finally it defines the physical properties of the tissue providing biomechanical cues to modulate cell behavior (reviewed by (Lu *et al.*, 2012)).

Tenascin-C is a large hexameric extracellular glycoprotein, discovered nearly 30 years ago by a number of independent laboratories (Bourdon *et al.*, 1983; Chiquet and Fambrough, 1984; Erickson and Inglesias, 1984; Grumet *et al.*, 1985). Identified as the antigen to monoclonal antibody 81C6, raised against glial fibrillary acidic protein (GFAP)-positive glioma cells (Erickson and Taylor, 1987), high levels of tenascin-C were detected in the tumor stroma and around the vasculature of glioma tissue (Bourdon *et al.*, 1983). Indeed, tenascin-C can be purified from human glioblastoma cultures, with yields reported up to 10 mg from 1 L of medium (Aukhil *et al.*, 1990). This specific induction of tenascin-C expression in glioma tissue, highlighted its potential use as a much needed tumor specific marker and only 5 years later, the antibody 81C6 was shown to specifically deliver cytotoxic radioisotopes to subcutaneous human glioma xenografts in mice or intracranial human glioma xenografts in rats with significant therapeutic effect (Lee *et al.*, 1988a; Lee *et al.*, 1988b). Since then, the distinct pattern of expression of tenascin-C has become increasingly well characterized and its use both as a diagnostic and prognostic marker for a number of different cancers has become increasingly sophisticated. Moreover, promising results in phase II clinical trials targeting tenascin-C as a unique therapeutic modality to treat some types of tumor have been reported. Here we review the recent advances in this field, highlighting new ideas that have emerged about the expression of tenascin-C in cancer, in addition to what is known about how this protein contributes to tumorigenesis from within the extracellular matrix.

## 1.1   Tenascin-C Structure

The human *tenascin-C* gene is located on the antisense strand of chromosome 9q33.1, flanked by the *DEC1* and *TNFSF8* genes, separated by ~23 kb and ~90 kb of intergenic sequences, respectively. The *tenascin-C* gene is relatively large, spanning 97,680 nucleotides and comprising 30 exons (Gherzi *et al.*, 1995; Mighell *et al.*, 1997; Sriramarao and Bourdon, 1993). The first exon is untranslated, with translation starting in exon 2. The exons range in size from 90 to 1410 nucleotides and the introns from 578 to

26,827 nucleotides. The mature mRNA transcript is 8150 nucleotides long, and the entire protein-coding region comprises 7500 nucleotides (Goh *et al.*, 2010). This RNA encodes a protein of a maximal length of 2385 amino acids (Hancox *et al.*, 2009; Jones *et al.*, 1989; Pas *et al.*, 2006).

The tenascin-C protein comprises a number of distinct structural domains. The N-terminal stretch of 110 residues is unique to tenascin-C and is followed by a short heptad repeat region. The adjacent epidermal growth factor (EGF)-like repeats, of which there are 14.5 in human tenascin-C, are 30 to 50 amino acids long and each contain six cysteine residues that mediate intrachain disulfide bonds. Next to these modules lie up to 17 fibronectin type III like domains (TNIII), which are ~90 amino acids long each and form two sheets of seven antiparallel β-strands. The number of TNIII domains is generated by alternative splicing; at least nine different TNIII domains are differentially included or excluded by RNA splicing. Finally, the C-terminal fibrinogen-like globular (FBG) domain is 210 amino acids long and forms intrachain disulfide bonds (Figure 1A). Tenascin-C possesses 23 potential glycosylation sites, two in the heptad region, two in the EGF repeats, 18 in the TNIII repeats and one in the FBG domain. Tenascin-C purified from human glioma cells is glycosylated (Taylor *et al.*, 1989) and this modification, together with alternative splicing, determines the molecular weight of the tenascin-C monomer that can range between 190 and 330 kDa.

Tenascin-C monomers are assembled into a hexameric form commonly called a hexabrachion (Figure 1B). The molecular weight of the hexamer was calculated to be $1.9 \times 10^6$ Da by sedimentation equilibrium analysis and by electrophoresis on non-reducing agarose gels (Taylor *et al.*, 1989). Pulse chase data indicate that nascent tenascin-C polypeptides rapidly assemble into hexamers intracellularly, even prior to completion of translation, and that this is followed by slower transport to the Golgi before secretion (Redick and Schwarzbauer, 1995). Hexamer assembly comprises a sequential two-step process. Trimerization is first mediated by the formation of a parallel three stranded α-helical coiled coil by sequences in the heptad repeats between alanine 114 and glutamine 139. This is followed by the connection of two trimers by sequences N-terminal to the heptad repeats (Kammerer *et al.*, 1998). Cysteine residues flanking this region are also important in tenascin-C multimerization: mutation of cysteine 64 abolishes trimer dimerization (Luczak *et al.*, 1998) and cysteines 111 and 113 are thought to further stabilize native tenascin-C by mediating interchain disulfide bonds (Kammerer *et al.*, 1998). Secreted hexameric tenascin-C can then be further assembled into a 3D matrix at the cell surface, creating a dense pericellular localization of fibrillar tenascin-C (Chung and Erickson, 1997; Chung et al., 1995).

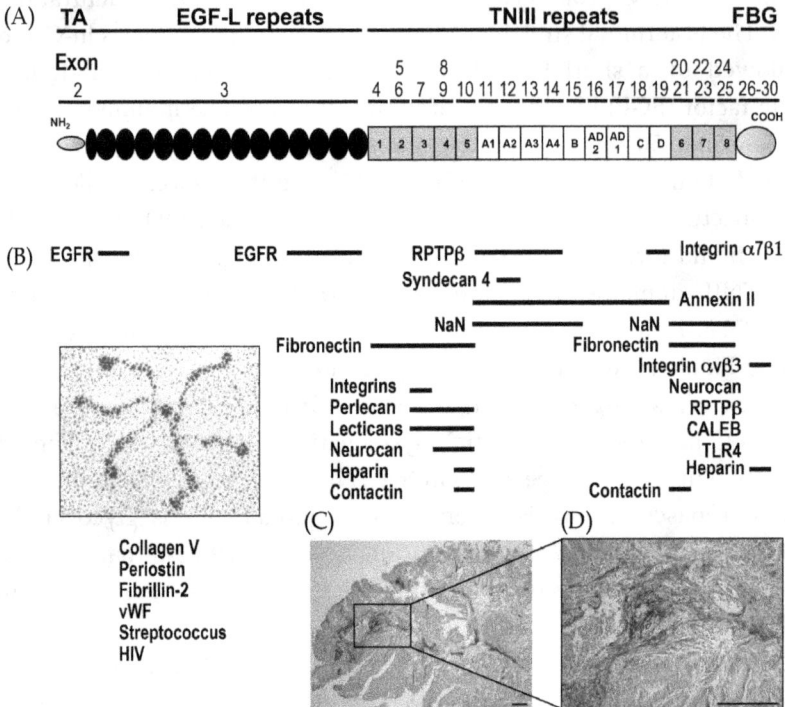

**Figure 1: Tenascin-C structure and expression in the tumor stroma.** (A) The exon/intron structure of the human tenascin-C gene and the organization into the different protein domains (based on analysis of sequence entries in the EMBL data bank). The multimodular organization of tenascin-C protein is shown comprising four distinct domains: an assembly domain (TA), a series of epidermal growth factor-like repeats (EGF-L), a series of fibronectin type III-like repeats (TNIII), and a C-terminal fibrinogen-like globe (FBG). Constitutively expressed TNIII repeats (1-8) are n in grey and alternatively spliced TNIII repeats (A1-D) in white. Molecules that bind to each domain of tenascin-C are also shown. (B) The appearance of purified tenascin-C protein as a hexamer upon electron microscopy. Image modified from (Midwood and Orend, 2009) and with courtesy to R. Chiquet-Ehrismann. (C, D) Tenascin-C in human colorectal cancer tissue visualized by immunohistochemistry using antibody B28-13. Scale bars = 200 μm.

## 1.2    Tenascin-C Expression in Tumors

Highly expressed during development, tenascin-C synthesis is down regulated postnatally and little or no tenascin-C is detected in most healthy adult tissues. It is transiently re-expressed upon tissue injury, but only for the duration of tissue repair (reviewed in (Midwood and Orend, 2009; Udalova *et al.*, 2011).

Tenascin-C is also highly expressed in glioma tissue, as originally observed in 1983, as well as in other types of cancer, but here expression persists throughout disease. Most malignant solid tumors exhibit high levels of tenascin-C including brain, breast, uterus, ovaries, prostate, pancreas, colon, stomach, mouth, larynx, lung, liver, kidney, bladder, skin and bone cancers, as well as cancers of soft tissues, and lymphomas. These data were extensively reviewed in 2006 and a detailed list of the expression of tenascin-C in tumors up to that point can be found in (Orend and Chiquet-Ehrismann, 2006). The majority of these reports, and further studies in the last 8 years, have examined tenascin-C protein expression histologically. In many cases increased tenascin-C expression in the tumor stroma was observed (for example Figure 1C, D). Moreover, in cancers such as breast cancer, glioma, lung carcinoma and osteosarcoma, high tenascin-C expression correlated with low survival rates. Table 1 highlights cancers for which high stromal tenascin-C expression correlates with advanced disease activity or poor patient prognosis.

However, expression of tenascin-C is not universally associated with poor prognosis. For example, no correlation with clinical history or neurological function in pediatric supratentorial glioblastoma multiforme could be found (Germano *et al.*, 2000). Likewise there appears to be no correlation between stromal expression of tenascin-C and tumor stage or prognosis in stomach adenocarcinoma (Zirbes *et al.*, 1999), nor with invasion, metastasis or survival in gastric carcinoma (Ikeda *et al.*, 1995; Ilunga and Iriyama, 1995). Tenascin-C is not a predictor for survival in oral and pharyngeal squamous cell carcinomas (Atula *et al.*, 2003), nor does it correlate with survival, clinical stage or metastasis in pancreatic carcinoma (Juuti *et al.*, 2004). Furthermore, poor prognosis has been reported for cases of cervical carcinoma that exhibited no staining of stromal tenascin-C (Pilch *et al.*, 1999). Moreover, opposing data have emerged from independent studies of the same type of cancer. In contrast to studies that report high tenascin-C expression correlating with a low survival prognosis in breast cell carcinoma (see Table 1), other studies found no corre-

| Tumor type | Correlation of tenascin-C expression | References |
|---|---|---|
| Adrenal pheochromocytoma | Prediction of aggressiveness | (Salmenkivi et al., 2001) |
| Astrocytoma | Correlation with higher tumor grade and proliferation. | (Zagzag et al., 1995) |
| | Correlation with degree of histological malignancy | (Higuchi et al., 1993) |
| Astrocytoma, oligodendrocytoma, glioblastoma | Elevated compared to normal tissue | (Brellier et al., 2011b) |
| Bladder carcinoma | Correlation with shorter survival | (Brunner et al., 2004) |
| Breast carcinoma | Associated with malignancy | (Mackie et al., 1987) |
| | Correlation with vascular grade and early invasion | (Tokes et al., 1999) (Jahkola et al., 1998a) |
| | In axillary node negative cases, expression at invasion boarder serves as prognostic factor for local recurrence | (Jahkola et al., 1998b) |
| | Correlation with lymph node metastasis and poor outcome | (Ishihara et al., 1995) |
| | Inverse correlation with receptor status, correlation with lymph node status and tumor grade, marker for negative prognostic value in invasive cancer | (Ioachim et al., 2002) |
| | Correlation with shorter survival of tamoxifen-treated patients with estrogen-positive breast cancer | (Helleman et al., 2008) |
| | Correlates with aggressiveness of lung metastases | (Oskarsson et al., 2011; Tavazoie et al., 2008) |
| Breast carcinoma, adenoses, fibroadenoma | Diagnosis of malignant disease and prediction of invasive potential of premalignant lesions | (Goepel et al., 2000) |

| | | |
|---|---|---|
| Colorectal carcinoma | Correlation with advanced stage and shorter survival | (Sis et al., 2004) |
| | Correlation with progression and metastatic spread | (Emoto et al., 2001) |
| | Correlation with lymph node metastasis | (Riedl et al., 1992) |
| | Correlation with poor prognosis | (Sugawara et al., 1991) |
| Ependymoma | Prediction of recurrence | (Korshunov et al., 2000) |
| | Correlation with decreased progression-free survival | (Zamecnik et al., 2004) |
| Endometrial carcinoma | Correlation with metastasis, muscle and vascular invasion | (Doi et al., 1996) |
| Giant cell tumors of bone | Predictive of local recurrence and metastasis | (Pazzaglia et al., 2010) |
| Glioma | Correlation with shorter survival | (Leins et al., 2003) |
| | Prognostic for early tumor recurrence | (Herold-Mende et al., 2002) |
| | Correlation with macrophagic/microglial infiltration | (Kulla et al., 2000) |
| | Correlation with vascular proliferation and malignancy | (Oz et al., 2000) |
| Insulinoma | Correlation of high tenascin-C expression with lymph node and liver metastasis | (Saupe et al., 2013) |
| Laryngeal and hypopharyngeal carcinoma | Correlation with metastases, tumor recurrence and lethality | (Juhasz et al., 2000) |
| Medulloblastoma | Correlation with poor prognosis | (Korshunov et al., 1999) |
| Non-small cell lung carcinoma | Correlates with microvessel density and shorter survival | (Ishiwata et al., 2005) |
| | Predicts malignancy | (Kahn et al., 2012) |
| Oral squamous carcinoma | Indicative of poor prognosis | (Lyons and Jones, 2007) |
| | Predicts poor prognosis and survival | (Wang et al., 2010b) |

| Osteosarcoma | Correlation with metastasis and poor survival | (Tanaka et al., 2000) |
|---|---|---|
| Papilla Vater carcinoma | Correlation with poor prognosis | (Vaidya et al., 1996) |
| Peripheral nerve sheath tumor | Distinguishes malignant from benign tumors | (Dugu et al., 2010) |
| Pleural mesothelioma | Correlation with malignancy and shorter survival | (Kaarteenaho-Wiik et al., 2003) |
| Primary melanoma | Absence of tenascin-C at invasion front correlates with lower risk for metastasis | (Ilmonen et al., 2004) |
| Prostate carcinoma | Little staining in high grade tumors but in well and moderately differentiated staining correlates with tumor progression | (Xue et al., 1998a; Xue et al., 1998b) |
| Renal cell carcinoma (clear cell) | Associated with higher stage and nuclear grade and lower survival and predictor of metastatic potential | (Ohno et al., 2008) |
| Salivary gland tumors | Correlation with metastasis | (Felix et al., 2004) |
| | Marker for recurrent disease in benign tumors | (Karja et al., 1995) |
| Urothelial carcinoma | Correlation with grade, stage and proliferative activity and shorter survival | (Ioachim et al., 2005) |
| | Expression higher in more aggressive micropapillary variant | (Ishii et al., 2011) |
| Vulvar carcinoma | Marker of malignancy and correlation with inflammation | (Goepel et al., 2003) |

**Table 1:** Stromal expression of tenascin-C protein as a diagnostic or prognostic marker of cancer.

lation between tenascin-C expression and prognostic factors such as p53, Ki-67 and estrogen receptor status (Tokes *et al.*, 1999), nor with long term survival (Iskaros *et al.*, 1998; Melis *et al.*, 1997). Some studies have even reported a positive correlation of tenascin-C expression with relapse free and overall survival (Suwiwat *et al.*, 2004) and better prognosis (Shoji *et al.*, 1993) in breast cancer patients. The expression and role of tenascin-C in breast cancer has recently been reviewed (Guttery *et al.*, 2010b). Likewise whilst some data show tenascin-C to be predictive of poor prognosis and shorter survival in colorectal cancer (Sis *et al.*, 2004; Sugawara *et al.*, 1991), other data show tenascin-C correlates with better long-term survival (Iskaros *et al.*, 1997). The reason for these differences is not clear and may depend on patient sampling and methods of disease assessment. What is clear is that the link between tenascin-C expression and each individual cancer is not always a straightforward or linear relationship. Indeed, in some cancers, whilst tenascin-C expression does not correlate with any clinical parameter, it is significantly linked to a specific aspect of tumor cell biology. For example, in chondyloma and intraepithelial neoplasias, there is no link between tenascin-C expression in the tumor stroma and hyperplasia but it was positively associated with inflammation (Pollanen *et al.*, 1996). Similarly, tenascin-C has been shown to be a reliable marker for epithelial proliferation in endometrial adenocarcinoma (Vollmer *et al.*, 1990) and to associate with tumor cell proliferation in adenoid cystic carcinoma (Shintani *et al.*, 1997).

Interestingly, in squamous cell lung carcinoma, in addition to tenascin-C staining in the extracellular matrix of the tumor stroma, intracellular tenascin-C was also reported (Soini *et al.*, 1993) suggesting that tumor cells constitute a cellular source of tenascin-C. In fibrohistiocytic tumors, an increase in cytoplasmic staining in tumor cells and a decrease in extracellular staining was observed in malignant disease (Franchi and Santucci, 1996). The significance of this intracellular accumulation of tenascin-C is not clear, nor is it known whether this effect is specific to tenascin-C or whether it reflects a global defect in tumor cell secretion with approaching malignancy.

In addition to the elevated tenascin-C protein expression reported in the tumor stroma, high levels of tenascin-C have been detected in the serum of patients with cancers including stage IV melanoma (Burchardt *et al.*, 2003), soft tissue carcinoma and squamous cell carcinoma. In these patients tenascin-C levels did not correlate with tumor burden (Schenk *et al.*, 1999; Schenk *et al.*, 1995). However, serum levels of tenascin-C were specifically elevated in head and neck squamous cell carcinoma at higher tumor stages and in recurrent disease (Pauli *et al.*, 2002) and in colorectal cancer serum levels did correlate with total tumor burden and metastatic disease (Riedl *et al.*, 1995). Moreover, serum tenascin-C levels were elevated in the cerebrospinal fluid of patients with astrocytic cancer, but not with any other type of brain cancer, and correlated with both the tumor grade and tumor dissemination (Yoshida *et al.*, 1994). These data suggest, as one might expect, that circulating or soluble tenascin-C may provide some information about the ability of certain tumors to spread, rather than revealing the status of the primary tumor.

In addition to examination of tenascin-C protein in cancer, investigation of tenascin-C mRNA has highlighted a number of interesting points. Firstly, these data reveal that the tenascin-C within a tumor may derive from either the tumor cell, the neighbouring stromal cell or from both cell types. For example, in malignant and fibroadenomatosus tumors, elevated tenascin-C transcripts were observed in both tumor and epithelial cells (Lightner *et al.*, 1994). In chondyloma and intraepithelial neoplasias mRNA was found in basal epithelium and in fibroblasts (Pollanen *et al.*, 1996). In breast ductal carcinoma mRNA was detected in cancer cells and stromal cells but in scirrhous carcinoma tenascin-C mRNA was only expressed by stromal cells (Yoshida *et al.*, 1997). Secondly, tenascin-C transcript levels have also been shown to correlate with clinical outcome. For example, in oral squamous cell carcinoma high transcript levels correlated with lymph node metastasis (Nagata *et al.*, 2003), in colon adenoma and carcinoma a correlation between transcript levels and the depth of invasion and frequency of metastasis to the lymph node was noted (Hanamura *et al.*, 1997) and in oral tongue squamous cell carcinoma, high levels of tenascin-C mRNA extracted from paraffin embedded biopsy tissue was predictive of poor prognosis (Wang *et al.*, 2010b). Furthermore, tenascin-C expression is not limited to cells within the primary tumor site; reverse-transcriptase polymerase chain reaction (RT-PCR) of RNA isolated from circulating tumor cells in patients with grade I and II colorectal cancer shows a positive correlation between tenascin-C and disease prognosis (Gazzaniga *et al.*, 2005).

More recently, array technology has been used to define tumor specific gene signatures, which frequently contain tenascin-C. Table 2 lists the tumors for which this type of analysis has been performed. In some cases total gene expression in biopsies of the primary tumor was assessed and a unique cluster of genes differentially expressed in the tumor com-

| Tumor type | Gene signature | Clinical use | Reference |
|---|---|---|---|
| Astrocytoma | Of 26 ECM specific genes, tenascin-C, brevican, neurocan & phosphoglycan were elevated | Correlated with an invasive phenotype in grade II tumors | (Varga et al., 2012) |
| Breast cancer | One of 95 genes linked to lung metastasis (48 overexpressed and 47 underexpressed), tenascin-C was elevated | Contributes to metastasis to the lung after xenograft in nude mice | (Minn et al., 2005) |
| | One of 6 ECM related genes upregulated: collagen 1A1, fibronectin, lysyl oxidase, SPARC, TIMP3 and tenascin-C | Associated with resistance to tamoxifen | (Helleman et al., 2008) |
| Giant cell tumors of bone | Of 109 differentially expressed genes that correlated with prognosis, tenascin-C was the most significant prognostic biological marker | Predictive for local recurrence and metastasis (4- and 8 fold increased risk respectively) | (Pazzaglia et al., 2010) |
| Glioblastoma | One of a 38 gene consensus profile: 31 associated with poor prognosis (including tenascin-C) and 7 associated with better prognosis | Predictive for malignancy, associated tumor cell mesenchymal differentiation, angiogenesis and poor prognosis | (Colman et al., 2010) |
| | One of 31 validated genes | Associated with malignant glioma | (Persson et al., 2007) |
| Non-small cell lung carcinoma (endobronchial epithelial lining fluid) | Tenascin-C, [C-X-C motif] ligand 14, S100A9, and keratin 17 were upregulated compared to normal subjects and benign samples | Together with nodule size, tenascin-C positivity improved the prediction of malignancy | (Kahn et al., 2012) |
| Pulmonary adenocarcinoma | Genes (up): cyclin B1, polo-like kinase 1, tenascin-C, keratin 8, keratin 19, DAN topoisomerase 2A (down): caveolin 1 and 2, TIMP3, SOCS2 and 3, DOC2 and gravin | Present in tumor tissue but not normal lung tissue | (Wikman et al., 2002) |

**Table 2:** Gene expression signature of tenascin-C positive tumors; relation to diagnosis, prognosis and/or treatment response.

pared to normal tissue was identified. These genes, unrelated by function, family or pathway, were used to reliably predict disease stage or patient survival in giant tumors of bone (Pazzaglia *et al.*, 2010) or glioblastoma (Colman *et al.*, 2010). Profiling of total gene expression in the endobronchial epithelial lining fluid of non-small cell lung carcinoma also identified a gene signature including tenascin-C that was up-regulated in malignancy compared to normal or benign tumor tissue (Kahn *et al.*, 2012). In addition to serving as a marker for disease outcome, transcriptional analyses have also revealed that tenascin-C expression in the primary tumor may be indicative of how patients will respond to treatment. Helleman and colleagues showed that high tenascin-C expression in patients with estrogen receptor positive breast cancer correlated to shorter survival upon treatment with tamoxifen (Helleman *et al.*, 2008). This study provides the first hint that tenascin-C may be useful defining the most effective treatment for individual patients, as well as in disease diagnosis.

Global transcriptomic profiling has also been applied to stromal fibroblasts from areas of prostate cancer or from areas with benign hyperplasia either alone or co-cultured with the human prostate cancer cell line PC-3. Amongst the genes identified, tenascin-C was shown to be upregulated in tumor cells co-cultured with fibroblasts from the tumor stroma compared to non-cancerous fibroblasts (Reinertsen *et al.*, 2012). These data highlight the importance of the environment on tumor cell behaviour.

Further studies have focused their analysis on specific subsets of genes, comprising only those that code for extracellular matrix components, providing a more detailed descriptor of the tumor cell environment. For example, tenascin-C was one of 4 genes specifically upregulated in the astrocytoma extracellular matrix (Varga *et al.*, 2012). It was also one of 6 extracellular matrix genes uniquely expressed in the stroma of breast cancers (Helleman *et al.*, 2008). In both cases the expression of these gene sets were shown to be associated with an invasive cell phenotype and thus reveal the content of an extracellular matrix that is particularly permissive to tumor metastasis. These data also emphasize the fact that no extracellular matrix protein exists in isolation and suggest that, for those tumors where no clear association with a single molecule has been demonstrated, analysis of a number of molecules may be a more reliable indicator of disease malignancy or outcome. It would be interesting to perform a global assessment of these extracellular matrix signatures in further cancer types to define if a single unifying environment promotes the metastasis of distinct tumor types or if different tumors require tailor made extracellular matrices in order to disseminate.

An elegant series of recent papers has begun to address this question. Their data reveal that metastasis of the same tumor type to different secondary sites is driven by very different molecular mechanisms. Using whole genome derived primer sets, 95 genes were identified that were specifically associated with breast cancer cells that possessed high potential to metastasize to the lungs in nude mice, compared to cells with a low metastatic potential (Minn *et al.*, 2005). This gene set was largely distinct from the gene-expression signature of the same parental breast cancer cell lines that exhibit high potential to metastasize to the brain (Bos *et al.*, 2009) or to bone (Kang *et al.*, 2003) in nude mice. Amongst these gene sets, tenascin-C was specifically enriched in those breast cancer cells that spread to the lungs, but not to either the brain or bone. Most recently, Oskarsson and colleagues confirmed the relevance of these data in human breast cancer. They showed that a high level of tenascin-C in the primary breast tumor was specifically associated with a shorter time to lung relapse (median time from primary tumor diagnosis to lung metastasis was 24 months in cases with high expression of tenascin-C versus 56 months in cases with low tenascin-C). They also showed that tenascin-C expression was particularly high at the invasive edge of metastatic lung nodules and that high tenascin-C expression at this site predicted poor overall survival (median time from metastasis diagnosis to death was 7 months in cases with high tenascin-C expression and 34 months for cases with low tenascin-C). These data highlight the importance of the extracellular matrix not only in the growth of the primary tumor but also in driving tumor cell metastasis to specific secondary sites. This paper went on to demonstrate that cancer cell derived tenascin-C was required for survival of the lung metastasis, until stromal tenascin-C could be synthesized as the major source in the secondary lung site (Oskarsson *et al.*, 2011). The mechanism by which tenascin-C promotes tumor cell survival is discussed further in section 3.3 below.

Global analysis of tumor cell attributes has also extended to other 'omic approaches. miRNA profiling revealed lost expression of miR355 in aggressive breast cancer that metastasizes to the lung. Tenascin-C was identified as one of the genes down regulated by this tumor suppressor miR, providing some mechanistic insight into why high levels of tenascin-C are observed in malignant breast cancers (Tavazoie *et al.*, 2008). Proteomic analysis of normal and transformed mammary epithelial cells grown in 3D culture systems also identified tenascin-C as a mediator of tumor progression (O'Brien *et al.*, 2011). Laser capture micro-dissection was used to isolate vessels from clinical samples of invasive ductal carcinoma and the proteomic profile of this tissue compared to patient matched adjacent non-malignant breast tissue. These data show elevated tenascin-C in malignant vessels, amongst a list of 29 differentially expressed genes that could predict survival in independent sets of microarray data from breast cancer patients (Hill *et al.*, 2011). Furthermore, high throughput screening of 204 proteins using multiplexed immunoassays identified 11 analytes in the blood, including tenascin-C, that could distinguish women with ovarian cancer from those with benign conditions with 90% specificity and sensitivity (Amonkar *et al.*, 2009). These data may offer a non-invasive means to screen for malignant ovarian cancer, if validated in further blind studies.

Finally, investigation into the genetic contribution to the risk of developing breast cancer, using a wistar rat model, has identified a mammary cancer susceptibility locus. Fine mapping pinpointed a region of ~176 kb on chromosome 5 and showed that the WKy allele at locus Mcs5c reduces carcinoma multiplicity after 7,12-dimethylben-[α]anthracene exposure. This region itself is gene poor and thought to mediate this effect by regulation of genes outside the locus. One candidate found within this locus is tenascin-C; tenascin-C expression is reduced in the thymus and ovarian tissues of Mcs5c WKy homozygous rats compared to controls (Veillet *et al.*, 2011).

## 1.3    The Impact of Tenascin-C Splicing in Tumors

In addition to the reported increase in the overall level of tenascin-C in tumor tissues, changes in the way that tenascin-C is spliced also occur during tumorigenesis. Upon western blotting of basal cell carcinoma lysates, two distinct tenascin-C variants of 210 and 300 kDa were detected, in contrast to detection of only the larger variant in normal cultured human skin fibroblasts (Verstraeten *et al.*, 1992). Conversely, western, as well as northern, blotting showed that a high MW tenascin-C variant was more strongly expressed in hyperplastic and neoplastic breast compared to normal breast tissue (Borsi *et al.*, 1992). Interestingly, normal human articular chondrocytes exhibited a high ratio of small to large splice tenascin-C whereas chondrosarcoma cell lines possessed a low small to large splice ratio. Clinical chondrosarcoma specimens with a lower small to large splice variant ratio showed a trend towards decreased survival suggesting that the prognosis of these patients may be predicted by assessing the ratio of tenascin-C variants (Ghert *et al.*, 2001).

A number of studies have more precisely identified alternatively spliced TNIII repeats that are expressed in a cancer tissue-specific manner and these are summarized in Figure 2. Hindermann and colleagues used a probe spanning TNIII repeats A3, A4 and B to localize expression of tenascin-C variants containing these alternatively spliced domains by *in situ* hybridization in oral squamous cell carcinoma. No reactivity was observed in normal non-keratinized buccal mucosa but transcripts containing these repeats were found in carcinoma and moreover correlated with malignancy (Hindermann *et al.*, 1999). The same probe was used to demonstrate that transcripts with domains A3, A4 and B are specifically found at the invasive front in prostatic adenocarcinoma, despite uniform staining of the tumor stroma with antibodies recognizing repeats A1-A4 (Katenkamp *et al.*, 2004). These data imply that specific subsets of tumor cells synthesize cancer specific tenascin-C variants.

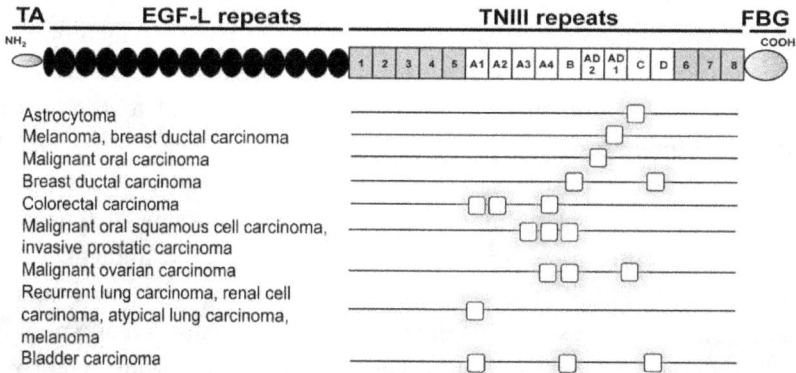

**Figure 2: Tumor specific TNIII domains.** Alternatively spliced repeats of tenascin-C that are reported to be up regulated or over represented in specific tumor types are shown.

Specific TNIII repeats have also been found to delineate malignancy or predict potential disease recurrence in a tumor specific manner. In ovarian cancer, larger transcripts containing TNIII A4, B and C are limited to malignant tumors (Wilson *et al.*, 1996). Repeat AD2 is not found in normal or premalignant mucosal samples but is found in a subset of patients with malignant oral mucosa (Mighell *et al.*, 1997). In non-small cell lung carcinoma, qRT-PCR analysis with primers for TNIIIA1 demonstrated that expression of isoforms containing this repeat correlated with tumor recurrence: patients with recurrent disease had an 18-fold increase in the expression of A1 positive isoforms compared to patients with non-recurrent disease (Parekh *et al.*, 2005). In colorectal cancer, extra repeat D is underrepresented in metastasizing cancers, whilst repeats A1, 2 and 4 are over expressed (Dueck *et al.*, 1999). The presence of extra repeat B and D correlates with the invasive phenotype of breast carcinoma by *in situ* hybridization (Adams *et al.*, 2002), and extra repeat B with Ki-67 levels in intraductal breast carcinoma and were found at the invasive front (Tsunoda *et al.*, 2003). In astrocytoma, repeat C is highly expressed in grade III tumors and in glioblastoma but not in breast, lung, gastric carcinoma or low grade astrocytoma (Carnemolla *et al.*, 1999). The presence of repeat C is also a marker of vascular proliferation in cavernoma (Viale *et al.*, 2002). An up regulation of repeats B and D in breast cancer (Adams *et al.*, 2002) and in ovarian cancer (Wilson *et al.*, 1996) has been reported.

The existence of tumor specific tenascin-C isoforms may explain why differences in tenascin-C expression have been observed in the same tumor types by different groups; data may be dependent on which probe or method of detection was used in analysis. Furthermore, these data have also provided insight into a potential functional role of tenascin-C domains in different tumors.

Hancox and colleagues identified how the presence of these extra repeats causes distinct cellular responses. Overexpression of tenascin-C variants containing either domain B or domains B plus D in breast cancer cell lines or normal fibroblasts promoted tumor cell proliferation and invasion compared to expression of small spliced variants. Overexpression of all domains of tenascin-C stimulated MMP-13 expression (Hancox *et al.*, 2009). These data demonstrate how specific tumor supporting functions can be assigned to individual spliced domains. This group also showed that repeats AD1 and AD2 are over represented in invasive breast carcinoma more frequently in women younger than 40 years old and that AD1 expression correlated with estrogen receptor negative, grade 3 tumors. Moreover, expression of variants containing domains B, D and AD1 stimulated tumor cell invasion and growth *in vitro* (Guttery *et al.*, 2010a). The effect of alternatively spliced TNIII domains on resistance to cytotoxic agents has also been examined. Using pancreatic cell cultures, Gong and colleagues showed that addition of a recombinant protein comprising TNIII repeats A-D suppressed gemcitabine induced cell toxicity via interaction with cell surface annexin A2. Ligation of annexin A2 by repeats A-D activated phosphatidylinositol 3-kinase, Akt and nuclear factor-kappaB signaling (Gong *et al.*, 2010). These data imply that alternatively spliced regions of tenascin-C may confer tumor cell survival upon delivery of cytotoxic drugs and provide a potential point of therapeutic intervention.

Indeed targeting tumors using antibodies raised against specific tenascin-C splice variants has been validated in a number of tumor types. The distribution of TNIII domains A1-D in urinary bladder carcinoma was assessed by immunohistochemical staining using domain specific antibodies and RT-PCR. Whilst a universal increase in large variant tenascin-C was observed in tumors of a higher grade, domains A1, B and / or D were restricted to invasive tumors and tumor vessels; repeats AD1 and C were rarely expressed (Berndt *et al.*, 2006). Phage display was subsequently used to generate antibodies specific for domains A1 and D. Both antibodies selectively accumulated at tumor sites in a U87 glioblastoma murine xenograft model but were rapidly cleared from other organs. Accumulation of antibodies to domain D was lower than that of antibodies to domain A1 and the former exhibited some non-specific localization to the intestine (Brack *et al.*, 2006). Based on these data, antibodies recognizing domain A1 have been further characterized; they are able to selectively stain tumor tissue, for example most Hodgkin and non-Hodgkin lymphomas (Schliemann *et al.*, 2009). The same authors report expression of A1 in renal cell carcinoma and atypical carcinoid of the lung (Berndt *et al.*, 2010), as well as primary cutaneous melanoma lesions, particularly in the basal lamina at the interface between epidermis and dermis (Frey *et al.*, 2011). In addition, vascular expression of A1, as well as domain C, has been reported in renal cell carcinoma (Galler *et al.*, 2012). Given the tumor specific pattern of tenascin-C splicing, antibodies targeting alternatively spliced tenascin-C domains, particularly repeat A1, are currently being used in clinical trials for the delivery of cytokines or therapeutic radionuclides to tumor sites in patients with cancer, whilst sparing unaffected organs. These studies are discussed in Chapter 4.

## 1.4   Tenascin-C: Form Versus Function in Tumors

Tenascin-C is assembled into a pericellular fibrillar matrix within the extracellular matrix. This 3D structure has quite different properties to soluble tenascin-C in terms of binding to other extracellular matrix proteins, affecting cell behaviour and defining the mechanical properties of the tissue (To and Midwood, 2011). The impact of the structural organization of tenascin-C within the tumor extracellular matrix has been investigated by Chen and colleagues. The assembly of tenascin-C into a dense fibrillar matrix was specifically observed in metastatic pancreatic cancers, compared to a less well organized matrix in benign tumors or healthy pancreatic tissue. Deposition of a fibrillar tenascin-C matrix by pancreatic tumor cells required co-culture of these cells with stromal fibroblasts, and purified fibrillar, but not soluble, tenascin-C reduced adhesion and promoted migration of tumor cell lines (Chen et al., 2009). These data highlight the importance of the structural organization of the extracellular matrix in defining the cell phenotype.

Tenascin-C in the extracellular matrix is also dynamically turned over. This can be mediated by degradation via the activity of numerous proteases including MMPs-1, -2, -3, -7, -9 and -19, or serine proteases; (reviewed in Udalova et al., 2011). Indeed in tumors, tenascin-C degradation products have been detected. Western blotting of tenascin-C purified from invasive colonic carcinomas displayed several low MW degradation products compared to that extracted from a human umbilical cord fibroblast cell line (Sakai et al., 1993). Subsets of patients with lung cancer demonstrated degradation of tenascin-C; and the presence of tenascin-C breakdown significantly correlated with metastasis to the lymph node and was thus proposed as a marker for metastatic potential (Kusagawa et al., 1998). Furthermore, in non-small lung cell carcinoma the presence of tenascin-C fragments was detected by western blotting tumor extracts and found in a subset of patients that exhibited recurrence of stage 1 disease. The absence of tenascin-C fragments was predictive of a good prognosis for lack of recurrence at 4 and 10 years (Cai et al., 2002). Finally, levels of tenascin-C isoforms containing TNIII domains B and C was analysed by ELISA in the urine of patients with urothelial carcinoma. Levels of both were increased as tumors progressed as did the presence of tenascin-C fragments (Richter et al., 2009). Proteolytic fragments of tenascin-C can be biologically active, often containing cryptic functions not present in full-length tenascin-C (To and Midwood, 2010).

In summary, existing data demonstrate a consistent up regulation of tenascin-C in a wide variety of tumors. However, these studies also highlight the complexities of associating tenascin-C expression with disease activity and prognosis. For some tumor types corroborative, independent data indicate that tenascin-C expression alone, or as part of a wider gene signature, may constitute a reliable marker for disease diagnosis and prognosis, most notably in glioblastomas. Further studies reveal that analysis of tenascin-C expression may indicate the most effective method of treating patients, for example subsets of breast cancer patients. Tenascin-C also appears to constitute a specific marker of tumor cells likely to metastasize to distinct secondary sites. Moreover, the precise form of tenascin-C expressed in each type of cancer may have a profound impact on tumor cell phenotype; the pattern of tenascin-C splicing, and the supramolecular assembly or degradation of tenascin-C may each contribute to disease progression.

# Chapter 2

# The Function of Tenascin-C in the Tumor Stroma

I n this chapter we discuss functional data that reveal what the purpose of tenascin-C in tumors may be by focusing on studies that have examined what this extracellular matrix glycoprotein is doing in the tumor stroma as well as at sites of metastatic colonization.

Tenascin-C is an extraordinarily pleiotrophic molecule. This functional plasticity is made possible by the multimodular structure of the molecule. Each domain of tenascin-C interacts with a number of specific matrix molecules and cell surface receptors (Table 3, Figure 1B). In this way, tenascin-C can influence tissue structure, modulate signals derived from other extracellular components, and signal directly to cells to affect cell phenotype.

## 2.1 Cell Adhesion, Proliferation and Survival

Tenascin-C has long been known to modulate cell adhesion, proliferation and survival. These effects, and the mechanisms by which they are mediated specifically in the context of tumor cell biology, are described in detail in several reviews (Chiquet-Ehrismann and Tucker, 2011; Orend and Chiquet-Ehrismann, 2006) and newer data are summarized below.

### 2.1.1 Tenascin-C Regulates Actin Dynamics and Impacts DKK1 Expression

Tenascin-C and fibronectin are frequently co-expressed in tumor tissue suggesting that they regulate cell behavior in the tumor microenvironment together as accomplices (reviewed in Van Obberghen-Schilling *et al.*, 2011b). This possibility is supported by the fact that tenascin-C counteracts the adhesive function of fibronectin in cell culture.

| Domain | Ligand | References |
|---|---|---|
| Full length tenascin-C | Fibronectin | (Chiquet-Ehrismann *et al.*, 1991) |
| | Collagen I – VI, IX | (Faissner *et al.*, 1990) |
| | Von Willebrand Factor | (Schaff *et al.*, 2010) |
| | SMOC1 | (Brellier *et al.*, 2011b) |
| | Periostin | (Kii *et al.*, 2010) |
| | Nidogen-2 | (Brellier *et al.*, 2011b) |
| | Fibrillin-2 | (Brinckmann *et al.*, 2010) |
| | Phosphoglycerate kinase 1 | (Brellier *et al.*, 2011b) |
| | Clusterin | (Brellier *et al.*, 2011b) |
| | Streptococcus | (Vollmer *et al.*, 2010) |
| | HIV-1 Env gp120 (V3 loop) | (Fouda *et al.*, 2013) |
| TA | Tenascin-C | (Kammerer *et al.*, 1998; Luczak *et al.*, 1998) |
| EGF-L 1-2 | EGFR | (Swindle *et al.*, 2001) |
| EGF-L 11-14 | EGFR | (Swindle *et al.*, 2001) |
| TNIII 3 | $\alpha v \beta 3$, $\alpha 2 \beta 1$ | (Sriramarao *et al.*, 1993) |
| | $\alpha v \beta 3$, $\alpha v \beta 6$ | (Prieto *et al.*, 1993) |
| | $\alpha v \beta 3$, $\alpha 9 \beta 1$, $\alpha v \beta 6$ | (Yokosaki *et al.*, 1996) |
| | $\alpha v \beta 1$ | (Probstmeier and Pesheva, 1999) |
| | $\alpha 8 \beta 1$ | (Denda *et al.*, 1998; Schnapp *et al.*, 1995) |
| TNIII 3-5 | Perlecan, lecticans | (Chung and Erickson, 1997; Day *et al.*, 2004) |
| TNIII 4-5 | Neurocan | (Rauch *et al.*, 2001) |
| TNIII 5-6 | Heparin | (Fischer *et al.*, 1995; Jang *et al.*, 2004; Weber *et al.*, 1995) |
| | Glypican | (Vaughan *et al.*, 1994) |
| TNIII 5 | Contactin | (Zisch *et al.*, 1992) |
| TNIII A1-A4 | RPTP$\beta$ | (Milev *et al.*, 1997) |
| TNIII A1-B | NaN | (Srinivasan *et al.*, 1998) |
| TNIII A1-D | Annexin II | (Chung and Erickson, 1994) |
| TNIII A2 | Syndecan-4 | (Saito *et al.*, 2007) |
| TNIII D | Integrin $\alpha 7 \beta 1$ | (Mercado *et al.*, 2004) |
| TNIII 6 | Contactin | (Zisch *et al.*, 1992) |
| TNIII 6-8 | NaN | (Srinivasan *et al.*, 1998) |
| FBG | Heparin | (Fischer *et al.*, 1995; Jang *et al.*, 2004; Weber *et al.*, 1995) |
| | Neurocan | (Rauch *et al.*, 2001) |
| | CALEB | (Schumacher *et al.*, 2001) |
| | Integrin $\alpha v \beta 3$ | (Yokoyama *et al.*, 2000) |
| | RPTP$\beta$ | (Milev *et al.*, 1997) |
| | TLR4 | (Midwood *et al.*, 2009) |

**Table 3:** Extracellular matrix proteins and cell surface receptors that interact with or are activated by tenascin-C

While fibronectin has long been known to promote cell adhesion, via activation of integrin $\alpha5\beta1$ signaling, assembly of focal adhesions and stabilization of actin filaments, tenascin-C specifically blocks the adhesion of cells to fibronectin (Chiquet-Ehrismann *et al.*, 1988; Murphy-Ullrich *et al.*, 1991; Spring *et al.*, 1989), and interferes with cell spreading, focal contact formation and actin stress fiber formation (Huang *et al.*, 2001; Orend *et al.*, 2003; Wenk *et al.*, 2000) and thus potentially counter balances strong cell adhesion to fibronectin *in vivo*.

Cells spread on fibronectin upon concomitant ligation of integrin $\alpha5\beta1$ and syndecan-4 by distinct sites in fibronectin (Bloom *et al.*, 1999; Tumova *et al.*, 2000; Woods and Couchman, 1994). During cell spreading focal adhesion formation precedes actin stress fiber formation, which also stimulates cell spreading. In tumor cells (including T98G, KRIB, MDA-MB 435 and J82) and in fibroblasts tenascin-C interferes with cell spreading, focal adhesion and actin stress fiber formation when cells are seeded on dishes coated consecutively with fibronectin and tenascin-C in comparison to cells seeded on fibronectin alone. Cell adhesion on a fibronectin/tenascin-C substratum was also blocked in CHO-B2 derivative cells, irrespective if they do not express fibronectin binding integrins or overexpress $\alpha5\beta1$ integrin, suggesting that $\alpha5\beta1$ integrin is probably not a direct tenascin-C target. However, cell spreading, focal adhesions and stress fiber formation can be restored by overexpression of syndecan-4, but not syndecan-1 or syndecan-2. Binding of tenascin-C was mapped to the three heparin binding sites (Hep) within fibronectin (Huang *et al.*, 2001; Ingham *et al.*, 2004). It is possible that binding to these three sites in fibronectin by tenascin-C has a huge impact on its 3D configuration and / or leads to an extensive coverage of fibronectin and masking of one or all cell binding sites in fibronectin by tenascin-C. The binding site within the second Hep site was further mapped to the 13th fibronectin type III repeat in fibronectin (FNIII13) (Huang *et al.*, 2001) which is known to bind syndecan-4 (Bloom *et al.*, 1999). Finally, a 20 amino acid peptide representing the cationic cradle in FNIII13, a sequence that is instrumental in syndecan-4 dependent cell spreading on fibronectin (Bloom *et al.*, 1999), counteracted tenascin-C-induced cell rounding suggesting that binding of tenascin-C occurs within FNIII13 (which occurred with a similar affinity as syndecan-4) (Huang *et al.*, 2001). In further support spreading of syndecan-4-null fibroblasts was unaffected if tenascin-C was incorporated in a fibrin-fibronectin matrix, while upon overexpression of syndecan-4 those cells behave the same way as wild type fibroblasts that fail to spread and form stress fibers in the presence of tenascin-C (Midwood *et al.*, 2004a). Altogether these results suggest an instrumental role of syndecan-4 in cell spreading on fibronectin that is impaired by tenascin-C by a mechanism that involves competition of tenascin-C with syndecan-4 binding to FNIII13. Competition with syndecan-4 binding to fibronectin has also been shown by fibulin-1 and appears to be a recurrent mechanism (Williams and Schwarzbauer, 2009).

Downstream of integrin α5β1/syndecan-4 signaling, tenascin-C leads to strongly reduced activation of FAK, tropomyosin-1 RNA levels and RhoA protein stability (Lange *et al.*, 2007; Lange *et al.*, 2008; Ruiz *et al.*, 2004). The FNIII13 domain of fibronectin as well as overexpression of syndesmos (providing a link to paxillin downstream of syndecan-4) is able to restore levels of phosphorylated FAK (p-FAK), RhoA and tropomyosin-1 (Lange *et al.*, 2008). Also upon overexpression of tropomyosin-1, expression and phosphorylation of FAK and paxillin as well as cell spreading, focal adhesion and actin stress fiber formation can be restored (Lange *et al.*, 2008; Ruiz *et al.*, 2004). Together these observations suggest that both polymerization into actin filaments (implicating RhoA), as well as stabilization of actin stress fibers (implicating tropomyosin-1) are impaired by tenascin-C by a mechanism involving inhibition of syndecan-4. Given that syndecan-4 is an important regulator of integrin α5β1 recycling and coordinates focal adhesion dynamics involving syntenin and Arf6 in cell migration (Morgan *et al.*, 2013) inhibition of syndecan-4 by tenascin-C may also impact on syndecan-4 regulated cell migration.

Through its impact on RhoA tenascin-C may affect biomechanics of tissues. NIH-3T3 fibroblasts cultured in a three-dimensional fibrin matrix containing fibronectin lack stress fibres and form actin-rich filopodia upon addition of tenascin-C to the matrix. This is accompanied by reduced RhoA activity. Upon activation of RhoA by LPA, spreading and stress fibers can be restored in the presence of tenascin-C. The same effect is observed upon overexpression of constitutively active RhoA (RhoA V14) in Rat1 fibroblasts. When RhoA activity was inhibited by C3 transferase upon treatment with LPA no stress fibers formed in the presence of tenascin-C, suggesting that tenascin-C blocks cell spreading and stress fiber formation by inhibition of RhoA activity (Wenk *et al.*, 2000). Tenascin-C also inhibited contraction of the fibrin-fibronectin matrix. The effect of reduced matrix contraction could be reversed by either stimulation with LPA or overexpression of constitutively active RhoA. Matrix contraction could be fully restored by synergistic treatment with LPA and phosphatase inhibitors preventing FAK dephosphorylation by tenascin-C suggesting that FAK is also a critical player (Midwood and Schwarzbauer, 2002). On a fibronectin/tenascin-C substratum RhoA protein levels were restored in T98G GBM cells upon blocking the proteasome (Lange *et al.*, 2007), upon adding a peptide derived from FNIII13 or upon overexpression of syndesmos (Lange *et al.*, 2008).

Interestingly tenascin-C induces cell rounding by a second mechanism, besides blocking of fibronectin binding to syndecan-4. Tenascin-C induces expression of EDNR-A, an endothelin-1 receptor. Upon blocking of EDNR-A with the specific inhibitor BQ123, cell spreading can be restored, as well as p-FAK, p-paxillin, RhoA and tropomyosin-1 protein levels (Lange *et al.*, 2007). In contrast, activation of a second type of endothelin-1 receptor (EDNR-B) by endothelin-1, abrogates cell rounding on fibronectin/tenascin-C and restores p-FAK, paxillin, RhoA and tropomyosin-1 expression. On the contrary, inhibition of EDNR-B by BQ788 restores EDNR-A dependent cell rounding on a fibronectin/tenascin-C substratum (Lange *et al.*, 2007). Thus the balance between activation of both EDNR receptors appears to regulate whether a fibronectin/tenascin-C substratum is anti-adhesive or allows cells to adhere and spread. This could be highly relevant for cell migration. In addition, these data demonstrate an important role of tenascin-C in impairing the function of molecules that are instrumental in cell spreading and migration such as FAK, paxillin, RhoA and tropomyosin-1.

Treatment with growth factors such as LPA and PDGF-BB can also cause cell spreading on fibronectin/tenascin-C by restoring p-FAK, p-paxillin, RhoA and tropomyosin-1 protein levels; this mechanism bypasses syndecan-4 signaling, as cell spreading can still be induced in MEF knockout for syndecan-4. Yet, spreading on a fibronectin/tenascin-C substratum induced by LPA/PDGF-BB is dependent on paxillin, as siRNA-mediated knockdown of paxillin hampered cell spreading (Lange *et al.*, 2008).

Altogether, in the tumor microenvironment tenascin-C may reduce strong cell adhesion to fibronectin by blocking syndecan-4 signaling. This mechanism appears to be superimposed by other signaling e.g. by signaling through ENDR-B or LPAR and PDGFR that counteracts cell rounding by tenascin-C. These data presumably can be extended to other signaling, which has not yet been revealed and demonstrate that integration of all signals (derived from transmembrane receptors such as growth factor receptors, integrins, syndecans and others) will determine the cell pheno-type in response to a tenascin-C substratum.

Recently, there were even other mechanisms described that alter the anti-adhesive properties of tenascin-C in cell culture in particular towards fibronectin. Proteolytic cleavage by Meprinβ creates a tenascin-C mole-cule that is impaired in oligomerization as well as in blocking cell adhe-sion to a fibronectin substratum. It was shown that T98G GBM cells spread equally well on a composite fibronectin substratum containing Meprinβ-cleaved tenascin-C as on fibronectin (Ambort *et al.*, 2010). In contrast to Meprinβ the gingipain family of cysteine proteases, expressed by the periodontopathogenic bacterium *Porphyromonas gingivalis*, degrad-ing extracellular matrix of periodontal tissues and leading to tissue de-struction and apoptosis, generated tenascin-C fragmented molecules that even enhanced cell rounding on fibronectin (Ruggiero *et al.*, 2013).

What impact does cell rounding by tenascin-C have on gene expres-sion and does this involve disruption of the actin cytoskeleton network by tenascin-C? It is well known that the polymerization state of actin has a huge impact on subcellular localisation of transcriptional regulators and gene transcription (Halder *et al.*, 2012; Olson and Nordheim, 2010). A comprehensive RNA profiling approach had been used to address how a tenascin-C containing substratum impacts on gene expression. The RNA expression profile of T98G cells was very different when cells were grown on fibronectin/tenascin-C in comparison to a fibronectin substratum (Ruiz *et al.*, 2004). Amongst the 373 differentially regulated genes, the largest and most diverse group of molecules specifically regulated by tenascin-C were genes encoding signal transduction molecules including EDNR-A, PDGFRα, c-fos and other genes that were increased by tenas-cin-C. On the contrary, a group of actin cytoskeleton-associated genes was noted to be down regulated by tenascin-C including tropomyosin-1, zyxin, dystrophin and cdc42 effector protein 3. Dickkopf-1 (DKK1), origi-nally identified as a Wnt signaling inhibitor was with 5-fold down regula-tion one of the most strongly repressed genes by tenascin-C (Ruiz *et al.*, 2004). Given that tenascin-C impairs actin stress fiber formation the ques-tion arises whether DKK1 expression is regulated by the tenascin-C spe-cific lack of actin stress fibers. Indeed, recently it was shown that disrup-tion of actin stress fibers by drugs such as latrunculin B or by a fibron-ectin/tenascin-C substratum led to very low DKK1 mRNA expression which was due to reduced DKK1 promoter activity. On the contrary, ac-tin stress fiber stabilization brought about by tropomyosin-1 and syndesmos over expression, respectively strikingly elevated DKK1 mRNA expression. Finally, in T98G cells where LPA had triggered actin stress fiber formation on the fibronectin/tenascin-C substratum DKK1 levels were determined and found to be restored to levels as on fibronectin. Yet, expression of a constitutive active RhoA molecule did not restore DKK1 expression on the fibronectin/tenascin-C substratum arguing for a mechanism where RhoA is not the main downstream target of LPA that affects DKK1 expression. Altogether these results demonstrate that tenascin-C regulates DKK1 gene expression through its effect on actin polymerization/stabilization and provides a first detailed glance on how an anti-adhesive tenascin-C substratum can regulate gene transcription through its impact on the actin polymerization state (Saupe et al., 2013). It will be interesting to identify the molecular mechanism that links actin stress fibers to transcription of DKK1. Potential candidates are MKL1 and YAP/TAZ that have been shown to relay the actin polymerization status (Dupont et al., 2011; Miralles et al., 2003) and regulate DKK1 expression (Seo et al., 2013), respectively (Figure 3).

DKK1 has also been shown to be downregulated by a stiffened collagen substratum in ovarian carcinoma cells mimicking matrix rigidity by a mechanism that led to stabilization of β-catenin and induction of MTP-MMP (MMP14) (Barbolina et al., 2012). Tenascin-C is frequently found in complex extracellular matrix networks, so called matrix tracks (reviewed in Midwood and Orend, 2009). Whether these tenascin-C matrix tracks are sites of enhanced tissue stiffness and potentially have an impact on DKK1 expression through tissue stiffness is possible and needs to be addressed in the future (Figure 3).

### 2.1.2 Tenascin-C Promotes Survival and Proliferation of Tumor Cells and Induces Cell Cycle Arrest in Anchorage Dependent Fibroblasts

Analysis of cell responses towards tenascin-C had revealed already in the early days of its discovery that tenascin-C increases proliferation in mammary tumor cells after serum depletion (Chiquet-Ehrismann et al., 1986). This observation was extended later by several laboratories (reviewed in Orend, 2005) who finally linked stimulation of proliferation by tenascin-C to inhibition of integrin α5β1/syndecan-4-dependent cell adhesion (Huang et al., 2001). In contrast to tumor cells, the anti-adhesive tenascin-C or fibronectin/tenascin-C substratum caused an anchorage-

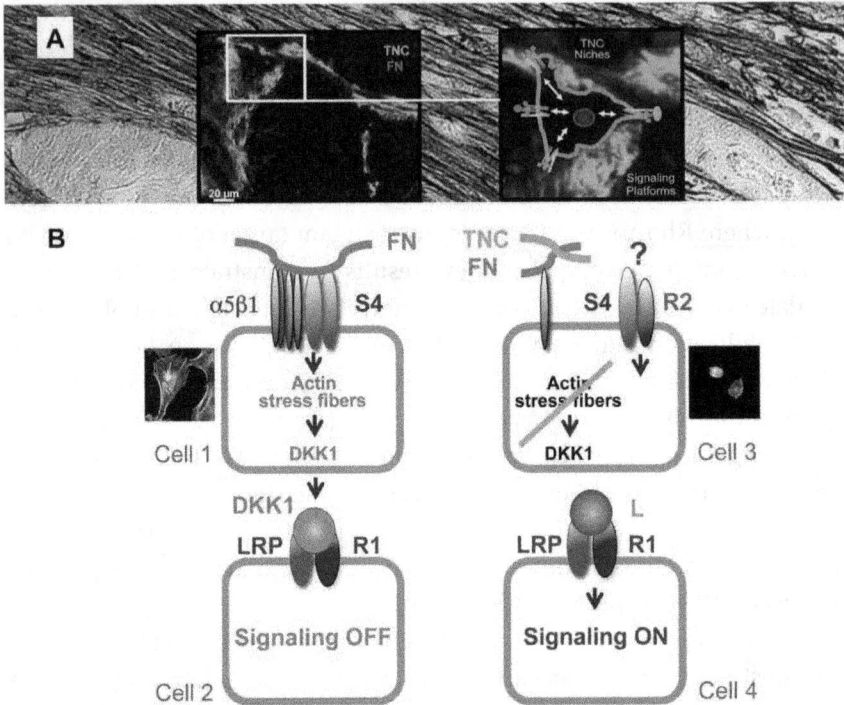

**Figure 3. Autocrine and paracrine impact of tenascin-C on Wnt signalling** A, Tenascin-C is found in extracellular matrix tracks, shown here for human colon cancer (background) (picture taken from Midwood *et al.*, 2011). Tenascin-C and fibronectin together form fibrillar networks into which cells are embedded. Cells integrate information from the microenvironment through specific signaling receptor platforms. This information is creating a signal that regulates gene expression and cell behaviour. B, Cell 1: upon binding to fibronectin through integrin α5β1 and syndecan-4 cells generate actin stress fibers and spread on fibronectin. This leads to expression of DKK1. Cell 2: upon secretion DKK1 can bind LRP6 (LRP) on an adjacent cell (paracrine mechanism) or on the same cell (autocrine mechanism). In the presence of Wnt (not depicted) LRP serves as a co-receptor for R1 (e.g. Frz, TGFβR, PDGFR, CTGF) and DKK1 appears to block this downstream signaling. Cell 3: Tenascin-C binds fibronectin and thus masks the cell binding site for syndecan-4 (S4) in fibronectin. In consequence no actin stress fibers are formed, cells remain rounded (actin staining picture on the far right) and DKK1 is not expressed. It is possible that syndecan-4 is now available as co-receptor for other syndecan-4 dependent receptor complexes (R2) (e.g. CXCR4/SDF1). Cell 4: Due to repression of DKK1, the tenascin-C microenvironment is characterized by low levels of DKK1 and thus facilitates LRP6 dependent signaling upon binding of the appropriate ligand (L) (e.g. TGBβ, PDGF).

dependent cell cycle arrest in several normal fibroblasts, human primary MRC-5, immortal rat REF52 and murine NIH3T3 fibroblasts that involved the cell cycle inhibitor p27Kip1 (Orend *et al.*, 2003).

When grown in a reconstituted basement membrane 3D microenvironment transformed non tumorigenic MCF-10A mammary epithelial cells formed three-dimensional polarized, growth-attenuated, multicellular acini, that were enveloped by a basement membrane. Addition of exogenous tenascin-C to this basement membrane microenvironment promoted cell proliferation and luminal filling by the MCF-10A cells which was due to an increased expression and signaling of c-met that could be blocked with a specific met inhibitor (Taraseviciute *et al.*, 2010). In another 3D growth condition where human breast cancer cells were grown as spheres, expression of tenascin-C by the tumor cells promoted their survival rather than their proliferation as was shown upon sh mediated tenascin-C knock down (Oskarsson *et al.*, 2011). Similar results had been obtained for neuroblastoma and melanoma oncospheres (Fukunaga-Kalabis *et al.*, 2010; Pezzolo *et al.*, 2011)(see below section 2.4)

To address the question whether the cellular source of tenascin-C plays a role in supporting tumor cell survival, breast cancer cells were engrafted by tail vein injection with a tenascin-C knock down (induced at different time points after cell grafting). It was shown that the tenascin-C knock down in the tumor cells lowered lung metastasis. As soon as the lung microenvironment expressed tenascin-C a tenascin-C knock down in the tumor cells did not impact on lung metastasis formation anymore. This result was interpreted as tenascin-C (provided by either the tumor or the stromal cells) being important for tumor cell survival in the lung (Oskarsson *et al.*, 2011). Yet it cannot be excluded that tenascin-C had also other effects such as promoting tumor cell adhesion to the endothelium, promoting tumor cell breaching through the endothelium and survival and/or proliferation in the lung parenchyma.

To address the contribution of host derived tenascin-C to lung metastasis 4T1 cells were intravenously grafted into mice and metastatic burden (area) was assessed in the presence and absence of host tenascin-C. Significantly less metastasis was seen in the tenascin-C knock out host supporting the notion that tenascin-C expressed by stromal cells plays a role in stimulating survival of metastasizing tumor cells or protecting them from apoptosis (O'Connell *et al.*, 2011). To further address which cells expressed molecules (including tenascin-C) in the lung that would promote metastasis of breast cancer cells, a mouse strain was used that had been engineered to selectively eliminate cells expressing S100A4 (comprising fibroblasts, myeloid and other cells). Ablation of S100A4 expressing cells was achieved by treating genetically engineered mice that expressed a thymidine kinase under control of S100A4 regulatory sequences with ganciclovir. Since tenascin-C was heavily expressed by S100A4 expressing cells and was largely reduced in lung tissue of mice with S100A4 depleted cells it is likely that these cells represent an important source of tenascin-C in the metastatic lung (O'Connell *et al.*, 2011). Yet other sources of tenascin-C may also be relevant.

Recently, in the well-established stochastic PNET/Rip1Tag2 model it was shown that transgenically expressed tenascin-C enhanced tumor cell survival and proliferation. In this model tenascin-C downregulated the Wnt inhibitor DKK1 suggesting that DKK1 and Wnt signaling might have an impact on tenascin-C promoted survival and proliferation. Yet, elevated DKK1 expression in KRIB osteosarcoma cells (engineered to overexpress DKK1) did not have an impact on survival nor proliferation in cell culture nor in grafted tumors (Saupe *et al.*, 2013).

Together these data reveal how tenascin-C can modulate cancer cell adhesion, survival and proliferation. These data are also discussed in more detail and in context of section 2.4 and chapter 3 below.

## 2.2   Immune Modulation

Our immune system is designed to protect us from invasion by pathogenic microbes and to help us repair tissue damage (Medzhitov and Janeway, 2002; Piccinini and Midwood, 2012). Immune cells constantly patrol the body on the alert for danger in the form of infectious organisms or tissue injury. These cells express pattern recognition receptors (PRRs) that sense conserved pathogenic molecules (pathogen associated molecular patterns [PAMPs]) or molecules that are generated by tissue injury (damage associated molecular patterns [DAMPs]). In response a program of inflammation is activated that will kill and engulf the invader and remove tissue debris. The immune system comprises two branches: innate and adaptive immunity. Innate immunity is the first line of defence that is activated immediately, or within hours, upon infection or injury and provides non-specific protection against any danger, mediated by the synthesis of pro-inflammatory factors including cytokines, proteases and reactive oxygen species. Adaptive immunity is antigen-specific and provides the host with a lifelong memory against reinfection with pathogens. This inflammatory program is inextricably linked to the tissue repair process. This is essential to rebuild the tissue lost as a result of the original injury and the damage caused by the inflammatory process itself and is mediated by the synthesis of a variety of growth factors that stimulate resident cells to proliferate, synthesize new extracellular matrix and re-vascularize the newly built tissue. Over time this tissue is remodeled and crosslinked so that it appears almost as good as new. Each of these phases of destruction (inflammation) and construction (repair) make up a highly orchestrated process that must be tightly regulated; for example too little inflammation or repair results in chronic, non-healing wounds, too much tissue deposition results in a variety of fibrotic diseases and over exuberant inflammation is the hallmark of a number of pathologies including auto-immune diseases, diabetes, atherosclerosis and indeed cancer (reviewed in Midwood *et al.*, 2004b).

Several inflammatory diseases, including inflammatory bowel disease, have been reported to increase the risk of cancer. Moreover, inflammation has long been associated with cancer. Tissue damage early in tumor development is thought to invoke a swift inflammatory response, causing the infiltration of immune cells including macrophages, dendritic cells, and T cells to the tumor microenvironment. Here myeloid cells synthesize high levels of pro-inflammatory mediators which have been shown to directly impact tumor cell biology. For example TNF enhances the growth and metastasis of a number of tumor types including skin, ovarian, pancreatic and bowel cancer, IL-6 has tumor growth and survival promoting activities in a wide range of cancer models and chemokine networks elaborated by these cells in the tumor have been shown to work together to facilitate tumor and immune cell migration, as well as angiogenesis, during primary disease, and to promote tumor cell egress during metastasis. Thus the inflammatory process is hijacked during the progression of cancer and used to the advantage of the tumor cell (reviewed in (Balkwill and Mantovani, 2012)). Furthermore, distinct types of lymphocyte activity have been linked with cancer progression. Acute tumor inflammation is characterized by a 'type 1' immune response. Mediated by a specific subset of CD4+ T cells, Th1 cells, this process is designed to fight the tumor. Th1 cells secrete high levels of interferon (IFN), a key weapon in this battle that can directly prevent tumor growth as well as activating anti-tumoral immunity, raising levels of histocompatibility genes, and activating macrophages and cytotoxic T cells. Chronic inflammation within the tumor is associated with a switch from a type 1 to a type 2 response. The hallmark of the type 2 response is the generation of an immunosuppressive environment that promotes tumor growth and aids metastasis. This is mediated by Th2 cells which persistently activate angiogenic and tissue remodeling programs, enhance cell survival and proliferation and promote immune evasion by the tumor. There is a large body of literature which demonstrates that re-setting the inflammatory axis to favour a Th1 response over a Th2 response can help provoke tumor cell death and cancer cell rejection (reviewed in Coussens *et al.*, 2013).

Tenascin-C expression has also long been associated with sites of inflammation in a wide variety of pathologies, and in the last two decades a number of inflammatory functions for this molecule have been described. These have been recently reviewed (Midwood and Orend, 2009; Udalova *et al.*, 2011) and are summarized in Table 4.

Tenascin-C has been shown to drive both innate and adaptive immune responses during tissue injury and infection (Midwood and Orend, 2009; Udalova *et al.*, 2011). Whilst its recently uncovered roles in pathogen defence (Piccinini and Midwood, 2012; Vollmer *et al.*, 2010) may not be relevant to the sterile inflammation that is the hallmark of the tumor environment, the ability of tenascin-C to induce the synthesis of several inflammatory cytokines, including TNF and IL-6, via activation of the cell surface receptors TLR4 (Liu *et al.*, 2012; Midwood *et al.*, 2009; Patel *et al.*, 2011) and α9 integrins (Asano *et al.*, 2013; Kanayama *et al.*, 2009), may contribute to disease progression by raising the levels of these tumorigenic cytokines in the tumor stroma.

Tenascin-C also drives the synthesis of chemokines such as IL-8 (Midwood *et al.*, 2009), thus stimulating the formation of high gradients of chemoattractants within the tumor stroma and potentially inducing further cell infiltration into the tumor site. Tenascin-C may additionally promote immune cell migration at tumors by directly interacting with cells. One study has shown that it supports lymphoid cell tethering to and invasion through complex extracellular matrices (Clark *et al.*, 1997). *In vivo*, inflammatory infiltrates during immune mediated hepatitis were less intense in tenascin-C null mice (El-Karef *et al.*, 2007) and tenascin-C null mice exhibit suppressed macrophage, but not neutrophil, invasion into cauterized corneas (Sumioka *et al.*, 2011). It is possible here that tenascin-C may act at a structural level by altering the conformation of the matrix to make it less restrictive and more migration permissive. Ultrastructural analysis of lymph nodes revealed that tenascin-C was deposited along the reticular fiber network forming putative 'footholds'

| Process | Function | References |
|---------|----------|-----------|
| Pathogen invasion | Supports streptococcal adhesion | (Vollmer *et al.*, 2010) |
| | Stimulates sustained cytokine translation upon bacterial infection by promoting the expression of miR-155 | (Piccinini and Midwood, 2012) |
| Thrombosis | Supports platelet adhesion and promotes platelet activation | (Schaff *et al.*, 2010) |
| Innate immunity | Stimulates TLR4-mediated cytokine synthesis | (Liu *et al.*, 2012; Midwood *et al.*, 2009; Patel *et al.*, 2011) |
| | Stimulates integrin mediated cytokine synthesis | (Kanayama *et al.*, 2009) |
| | Inhibits myeloid cell migration | (Loike *et al.*, 2001; Talts *et al.*, 1999) |
| | Stimulates macrophage migration | (Sumioka *et al.*, 2011) |
| | Stimulates hematopoiesis | (Klein *et al.*, 1993; Ohta *et al.*, 1998; Seiffert *et al.*, 1998) |
| | Promotes erythroid cell differentiation | (Tanaka *et al.*, 2009) |
| Adaptive immunity | Stimulates Th2 and B cell activation | (Kuhn and Mason, 1995; Nakahara *et al.*, 2006) |
| | Inhibits T cell activation | (Kuznetsova and Roberts, 2004) |
| | Promotes lymphocyte migration | (Clark *et al.*, 1997; El-Karef *et al.*, 2007; Sobocinski *et al.*, 2010) |
| | Limits T cell actin polymerization and migration | (Huang *et al.*, 2010) |
| | Drives Th17 cell polarization | (Kanayama *et al.*, 2011; Ruhmann *et al.*, 2012) |

**Table 4:** Overview of the inflammatory properties of tenascin-C

for T cell migration (Sobocinski *et al.*, 2010). In addition, tenascin-C has been shown to modulate the synthesis and activity of extracellular matrix degrading proteases *in vitro* and so in this way it may enable increased degration of extracellular matrix barriers to migration. Tenascin-C also directly influences cell phenotype, for example modulating polarity, focal adhesion turnover or cytoskeletal architecture, all processess that contribute to sucessful migration. Indeed tenascin-C may drive all of these events to bring about coordinated and efficient cell movement into and out of tumor sites (reviewed in (Midwood and Orend, 2009)).

However, it is important to note that these data supporting a role for tenascin-C in promoting immune cell migration contrast with data showing that tenascin-C limits immune cell migration. One study examining myeloid cell migration in a model system with a direct relevance to tumor cells showed that significantly higher levels of monocyte and macrophage migration were observed in the stroma of mammary tumors in tenascin-C null mice compared to wild type mice (Talts *et al.*, 1999). These data fit with *in vitro* studies showing that myeloid cells failed to effectively migrate through a matrix barrier containing tenascin-C, compared to matrices that did not contain tenascin-C (Loike *et al.*, 2001). More recently, Huang and colleagues demonstrated that tenascin-C mediated cross-talk between glioma cells and neighboring T cells is key for limiting T-cell migration within the brain. Here, CD3-positive T cells accumulated within blood vessels stained strongly with tenascin-C in glioma tissue and did not migrate into the brain tissue (Huang *et al.*, 2010). These data suggest an immune suppressive function of tenascin-C, whereby it prevents T cell mediated attack of the glioma.

Together these data exemplify the context specific nature of studies examining the role of tenascin-C, but do indicate that, in addition to direct modulation of tumor cell biology, tenascin-C may facilitate cancer progression by orchestrating the behaviour of tumor associated immune cells. Moreover, tenascin-C could comprise part of the molecular machinery that links inflammatory disease to susceptibility to developing cancer. Indeed, high circulating levels of tenascin-C are found in patients with inflammatory bowel disease (Riedl *et al.*, 2001) and this aspect of tenascin-C biology warrants further examination.

## 2.3   Angiogenesis

The growth of a tumor strongly depends on its supply of nutrients and oxygen. In the course of tumor development the angiogenic switch is considered a crucial event in promoting malignancy (Hanahan and Weinberg, 2011). The angiogenic switch is characterized by sprouting, new vessel formation, vessel maturation, and the recruitment of perivascular cells (Bergers and Benjamin, 2003; Hanahan and Weinberg, 2011). It can be triggered by pro-angiogenic growth factors and hypoxia as well as by the extracellular matrix of the tumor microenvironment (Bergers and Benjamin, 2003; Campbell *et al.*, 2010). The vasculature of a tumor often differs from vasculature in healthy tissues and is character-ized by chaotic vessels, a disorganized and disrupted basement mem-brane, incomplete pericyte coverage and leakiness (Shang *et al.*, 2012).

### 2.3.1   Tenascin-C as a Marker for Tumorigenic Blood Vessels

In several studies tenascin-C expression has been found to be preferen-tially localized around tumor blood vessels. In 86 gliomas, where tenas-cin-C expression increased with tumor malignancy, tenascin-C was strongly expressed around tumor blood vessels in glioblastoma grade IV (GBM). This was different in gliomas of WHO grade II and III with a re-duced frequency of tenascin-C lined blood vessels. In addition perivascu-lar tenascin-C staining in glioma grade II and III significantly correlated with a shorter disease free period (Herold-Mende *et al.*, 2002). Also Beh-rem and colleagues observed that GBM with strong perivascular tenas-cin-C staining contained more newly formed blood vessels than tumors with moderate or weak tenascin-C expression, as assessed by staining of CD105 microvessels (Behrem *et al.*, 2005). CD105 is defined as a prolifera-tion associated endothelial cell marker (Tanaka *et al.*, 2001). Furthermore in tissue samples from 63 patients with non-small cell lung cancer a corre-lation was found between serum tenascin-C and intratumoral vessel den-sity (Ishiwata *et al.*, 2005). In juvenile nasopharyngeal angiofibroma tenascin-C expression was also found around blood vessels where ex-pression correlated with vessel density, tumor stage and endothelial c-kit expression (Renkonen *et al.*, 2012).

Berndt and colleagues showed that in CD31 positive blood vessels of clear cell renal cell carcinoma and atypical carcinoids of the lung tenascin-C is localized at the extraluminal side of the basement membrane (Berndt *et al.*, 2010). By *in situ* hybridization tenascin-C mRNA was detected in astrocytoma tumor tissues in hyperplastic capillaries. Staining was ob-served lining the vascular lumen, indicating the presence of tenascin-C in endothelial cells. But other cells could also be a source of tenascin-C, as additional staining was observed in the walls of the vascular structures (Zagzag *et al.*, 1996). Indeed, data from Martina and colleagues showed that tenascin-C is expressed by pericytes in GBM but not by endothelial cells (Martina *et al.*, 2010).

Recently three studies using proteomic approaches have identified tenascin-C as a marker preferentially expressed in the vasculature of tumors or at the metastatic site. Borgia and colleagues used *in vivo* perfusion of biotin for labelling of vascular proteins. Four different tenascin-C isoforms (containing TNIII domains A1, A2, A4, B) have been identified as molecules, which were expressed in the vasculature of liver metastases in a syngeneic heterotopic model of colon cancer (Borgia *et al.*, 2009). Hill and colleagues used laser capture microdissection of microvessels of invasive ductal carcinoma and identified tenascin-C as one of the proteins overexpressed in tumor vessels in comparison to vessels from adjacent healthy tissue (Hill *et al.*, 2011). Similarly, by using laser capture microdissection and protein expression profiling tenascin-C was found to be exclusively expressed in tumor vessels of GBM but not in tissue with physiological angiogenesis (Mustafa *et al.*, 2012).

In summary, these data show that in a number of tumors tenascin-C specifically marks tumor blood vessels. Tenascin-C expression often correlates with higher tumor stage and increased blood vessel density, which argues for a role of tenascin-C in the tumor vasculature.

### 2.3.2    Tenascin-C Impacts on Endothelial Cell Behavior *in Vitro*

A number of studies showed that tenascin-C is able to modulate the behaviour of endothelial cells *in vitro*, including endothelial cell attachment and spreading, supporting migration and proliferation, as well as their sprouting. All these effects are known to be associated with angiogenesis and may contribute to the tumor angiogenesis promoting effect of tenascin-C.

Tenascin-C supported the switch from a non-angiogenic (resting) cobblestone phenotype to an angiogenic sprouting cord-forming phenotype in bovine aortic endothelial cells (BAEC) (Canfield and Schor, 1995). Schenk and colleagues showed that tenascin-C is exclusively expressed in the sprouts and cords of the sprouting but not in the resting BAEC. For the induction of sprouting by tenascin-C the growth factor basic fibroblast growth factor (bFGF) seems to be required. Furthermore the authors showed that the FBG domain of tenascin-C was responsible for the BAEC sprouting (Schenk *et al.*, 1999). The authors argued that the sprout-supporting effect of tenascin-C might be explained with the anti-adhesive effect of tenascin-C. However, conflicting observations have been reported concerning this issue. Whereas an anti-adhesive effect of tenascin-C on endothelial cells of different origin was shown (Ballard *et al.*, 2006; Sriramarao *et al.*, 1993) significant stimulation of tenascin-C on endothelial cell adhesion was reported by others (Delaney *et al.*, 2006; Zagzag *et al.*, 2002). These differences in results might reflect context dependent differences.

The anti-adhesive tenascin-C effect reported has been linked to a reduction in focal adhesions in endothelial cells (Murphy-Ullrich *et al.*, 1991). These authors showed that the TNIII A-D domain mediates the anti-adhesive effect, which can be reversed by blocking cell surface annexin II, a tenascin-C receptor (Chung *et al.*, 1996).

Despite its anti-adhesive and anti-spreading effect early upon cell plating, most endothelial cells eventually do attach and spread on tenascin-C after culture for longer periods of time. This cell attachment can be blocked with an RGD peptide (Bourdon and Ruoslahti, 1989). Endothelial cell attachment and spreading on tenascin-C was mediated by different tenascin-C cell surface receptors including annexin II (Chung and Erickson, 1994), $\alpha 2\beta 1$ and $\alpha v\beta 3$ integrins (Delaney *et al.*, 2006; Joshi *et al.*, 1993; Sriramarao and Bourdon, 1993). But in long-term assays endothelial cells secrete other extracellular matrix molecules such as fibronectin, and adhesion to fibronectin would be blocked with RGD peptides. Thus the described observation may be due to inhibiting adhesion to fibronectin with the RGD peptide rather than blocking the interaction with tenascin-C. Altogether these studies show that through different cell surface receptors adhesion and spreading of endothelial cells is modulated by tenascin-C, which could be crucial in tumor angiogenesis.

Tenascin-C was shown to enhance endothelial cell proliferation (Castellon *et al.*, 2002; Chung *et al.*, 1996; Delaney *et al.*, 2006) and, to promote endothelial cell migration (Ballard *et al.*, 2006; Castellon *et al.*, 2002; Chung *et al.*, 1996; Ishiwata *et al.*, 2005; Martina *et al.*, 2010; Zagzag *et al.*, 2002). This was demonstrated in different assays and with endothelial cells of different origin. Moreover it has been demonstrated that in the presence of tenascin-C there is increased sprouting and tube formation of endothelial cells (Castellon *et al.*, 2002; Martina *et al.*, 2010). The different effects of tenascin-C on endothelial cell behavior are summarized in Table 5.

### 2.3.3    Potential roles of Tenascin-C in Tumor Angiogenesis – Underlying Mechanism(s) and Signaling

There are several lines of evidence that tenascin-C can regulate tumor angiogenesis through enhancing pro-angiogenic signaling potentially by

| Assay | Experimental details | | | Cell line | Reference |
|---|---|---|---|---|---|
| | | ADHESION | | | |
| 10 min, 3hrs | Coating (10 µg/ml) | Compared to Collagen | Statistical difference, replicate experiments | CMEC | (Ballard et al., 2006) |
| 45 min | Coating (0.1 µg/ml) – for other ECMs higher conc. used | Compared to plastic, FN, VN (but less then LN, Coll) | No statistical difference if compared to plastic, 3 experiments | HDMEC | (Delaney et al., 2006) |
| 24h | Coating (no conc. mentioned) | FN/TNC 1:100 compared to FN/TNC 1:1 | Statistical difference, triplicate experiments | HUVEC | (Alves et al., 2011) |
| | | MIGRATION | | | |
| Wound healing assay, 48h | TNC (30 µg/ml) added to medium | Compared to plastic | No statistics provided, 1.8 fold increase, 7 experiments | GM7373 | (Chung et al., 1996) |
| Wound healing assay, 7d | TNC (40µg/ml) added to medium | Compared to IgG treatment | Statistical difference, 6 experiments | REC | (Castellon et al., 2002) |
| plating of EC aggregates on matrix, 22h | Coating of glass slides (100 µg/ml) | Compared to FN | Statistical difference, 3-10 observations | BREC | (Zagzag et al., 2002) |
| cell culture insert polyethylene terephthalate, underside of membrane coated, 5h | Coating (100 µg/ml) | Compared to FN | Statistical difference 4-10 observations | BREC | (Zagzag et al., 2002) |
| Boyden Chamber, reverse side coated, 6h | Coating (100 µg/ml) | Compared to BSA | Statistical difference, number of experiments not indicated | HUVEC | (Ishiwata et al., 2005) |

| | | | | | |
|---|---|---|---|---|---|
| migration into collagen gel ontop, medium with VEGF-A or PDGF-AB | Coating (10 µg/ml) | Compared to collagen | Statistical difference, 4 experiments | CMEC | (Ballard et al., 2006) |
| Time lapse, 10 h | Coating (200 ng FN or TNC in 72 well MicroWell Mini Trays + 20 µg/ml Collagen) | Coll/TNC compared to Coll/FN | Statistical differerence, 2 experiments | HUVEC | (Martina et al., 2010) |
| **TUBE FORMATION** | | | | | |
| Tube length, 48h | Coating (40 µg/ml) on BM matrix, or TNC added to the cells | Compared to no coating, LN, FN | Statistical difference, 3 experiments | REC | (Castellon et al., 2002) |
| Cumulative sprouts length, HUVEC spheroids in collagen gel, 48h | TNC (20 µg/ml) incorporated in the gel/secreted by HEK 293 spheroids | Compared to BSA/control cells | Statistical difference, 3 experiments | HUVEC | (Martina et al., 2010) |
| Number capillary like structures, HUVECs previously seeded for 24h on U373 cell derived matrix, seeded on matrigel for 16 h | α-TNC antibody incubation for 2h with U373 cell derived matrix | Compared to IgG treatment | Statistical difference, 3 experiments | HUVEC | (Alves et al., 2011) |

| Assay | Coating with TNC (concentration not specified) | Comparison | Result | Cell type | Reference |
|---|---|---|---|---|---|
| Number capillary like structures, HUVECs previously seeded for 24h on U373 cell derived matrix, seeded on matrigel for 16 h | Coating with TNC (concentration not specified) | TNC or FN/TNC compared to FN | No statistics provided, decrease in number of capillary like structures by approx. 4.5 or 1.6 respectively, comparing TNC or FN/TNC compared to FN | HUVEC | (Alves et al., 2011) |
| PROLIFERATION | | | | | |
| BrdU incorporation, 12h | TNC (30; 70; 100 µg/ml) added to medium | Compared to plastic | Statistical difference, at least 3 experiments | GM7373 BAEC | (Chung et al., 1996) |
| [3H] thymidine incorporation assay, 24h | TNC (40 - 100 µg/ml) added to medium | Compared to plastic | No statistics provided, approx. 1.6 fold increase, number of experiments not indicated | BAEC | (Chung et al., 1996) |
| Survival – secondary sprouting assay: number of cells in sprouting colonies 14 days after tube collapse | Coating (25 µg/ml) on BM matrix | Compared to no coating | Statistical difference, 2 experiments | REC | (Castellon et al., 2002) |
| MTS Assay (0.5% and 10% serum), 6 days | Coating (10 – 50 µg/ml) | Compared to plastic | No statistics provided, 20-40% increase, 2 experiments | REC | (Castellon et al., 2002) |

**Table 5:** Overview of tenascin-C effects on endothelial cells *in vitro*.

VEGFA. The initial study by Tanaka and colleagues suggests that tenascin-C supports melanoma angiogenesis by regulating the expression of VEGFA. After injection of melanoma cells (expressing tenascin-C) in immune compromised wild type and tenascin-C knock out (KO) mice tumors grown in KO mice were smaller and were less vascularized. Measuring the VEGFA content of the tumors by ELISA the authors observed a lower VEGFA content in tumors from the KO mice than those grown in wild type mice. Also in co-cultures with melanoma cells and the mesenchyme derived from either wild type or tenascin-C KO mice the authors measured a higher VEGFA level when the mice expressed tenascin-C (Tanaka et al., 2004). These data suggest that stromal cell derived tenascin-C contributes to tumor angiogenesis involving VEGFA (and presumably other factors). Tenascin-C expression was also seen to correlate with VEGFA levels in human cancers such as GBM (Behrem et al., 2005). In serum from non-small cell lung cancer patients tenascin-C levels correlated with the serum levels of VEGFA (Ishiwata et al., 2005). Moreover Sumioka and colleagues showed that occular fibroblasts derived from tenascin-C KO mice expressed less VEGFA than wild type fibroblasts which was associated with less neovascularisation of the cornea in tenascin-C KO mice (Sumioka et al., 2011). These are correlative data, yet how tenascin-C would impact on the expression of VEGFA is unknown.

Using surface plasmon resonance (Biacore) VEGFA binding to tenascin-C has been demonstrated (De Laporte et al., 2013; Saupe et al., 2013) which raises the possibility that a tenascin-C rich extracellular matrix may impact on VEGFA signaling. Moreover, not only VEGFA but also other growth factors including, CTGF, PDGF, TGFβ, IGF-BP and FGF were shown to bind to the fifth fibronectin type III repeat in tenascin-C (TNIII5) (De Laporte et al., 2013) and it is possible that this would apply to even other pro-angiogenic factors which has not been addressed yet.

Similarly, binding of VEGF to FNIII in fibronectin and tenascin-X has also been demonstrated and was linked to enhanced proliferation of endothelial cells and thus may represent a more common role of extracellular matrix to sequester and/or present VEGFA (Hynes, 2009; Ishitsuka et al., 2009; Wijelath et al., 2006). Whether the binding of growth factors to tenascin-C enhances their activity or blocks it needs to be addressed in the future. It is possible that a tenascin-C rich microenvironment contributes to the establishment of a gradient of pro-angiogenic growth factors that attracts endothelial cells and acts as a reservoir for pro-angiogenic growth factors (see below), which could be released upon activation of

MMPs or other extracellular matrix degrading enzymes, or that tenascin-C helps presenting growth factors to cell surface receptors similar to fibronectin (Hynes, 2009).

Tenascin-C has been demonstrated to upregulate the expression and function of other pro-angiogenic molecules such as PDGFRα (Lange *et al.*, 2008) and endothelin receptor EDNR-A (Lange *et al.*, 2007) in tumor cell lines derived from GBM, melanoma and urinary bladder carcinoma, respectively (reviewed in Orend, 2005). Whether these pathways have an impact on tenascin-C associated tumor angiogenesis remains to be seen.

To address the role(s) of tenascin-C in tumor vessels the well-established PNET/Rip1Tag2 insulinoma model of multi stage tumorigenesis (Hanahan, 1985) was used to generate the first stochastic tumor model with defined tenascin-C expression levels (Saupe *et al.*, 2013). In this study the authors had generated Rip1Tag2 mice with no and abundant tenascin-C expression (using tenascin-C KO mice and mice with transgenic overexpression of human tenascin-C encompassing all but the AD1 and AD2 domains). The authors observed that the extent of angiogenesis correlated with the tenascin-C copy number. The number of endothelial cells/vessel density was highest in tumors with expression of transgenic tenascin-C and lowest in tumors lacking tenascin-C. By isolation of pancreatic islets from tumor mice at 8 weeks of age when the angiogenic switch occurs it turned out that the number of islets that had undergone the angiogenic switch was higher in mice with transgenic tenascin-C than in mice with wild type tenascin-C and, lower in mice lacking tenascin-C in comparison to mice with wild type tenascin-C, altogether suggesting that tenascin-C promotes the angiogenic switch. Although tenascin-C promoted blood vessel formation these vessels were less functional when over expressing tenascin-C. In tumors expressing transgenic tenascin-C higher vessel leakiness was documented by increased fibrinogen staining outside blood vessels upon PBS perfusion as well as by a lowered number of pericyte covered blood vessels. Scanning electron micrographs of Mercox corrosion casts confirmed a highly aberrant vasculature in tumors with overexpressed transgenic tenascin-C since these tumor vessels were irregularly shaped, wider, discontinued, and bifurcated. In summary, this study has proven that tenascin-C is important in tumor angiogenesis by promoting the angiogenic switch leading to poorly functional blood vessels. This could have a negative impact on tumor growth and may promote metastasis (see below).

In addition to PDGF and EDNR-A signaling, Wnt signaling is another pathway regulating physiological and pathological angiogenesis (Dejana, 2010). Tenascin-C has been shown to down regulate the Wnt inhibitor DKK1 in several tumor cells including GBM (T98G), osteosarcoma (KRIB) and melanoma (MDAMB435) cell lines (Ruiz et al., 2004; Saupe et al., 2013) as well as in endothelial cells, pericytes and carcinoma associated fibroblasts (Saupe et al., 2013). Axin2 expression as readout for Wnt signaling was increased in tumor and endothelial cells but not in pericytes. In Rip1Tag2 tumors the expression levels of DKK1 inversely correlated with the tenascin-C copy number and were highest in tumors lacking tenascin-C and lowest in tumors that over expressed tenascin-C. At the same time Axin2 (the bona fide Wnt signaling target) as well as cyclin D1, CD44 and Slug, which are also transactivated by Wnt signaling, were elevated in tumors with transgenic tenascin-C.

How could DKK1 have an impact on angiogenesis? DKK1 was shown to bind LRP6 in several signaling complexes where LRP6 serves as co-receptor in canonical Wnt, PDGF, CTGF and TGFβ signaling (Ren et al., 2013), all pathways that had been shown to promote tumor angiogenesis. Thus, tenascin-C may create a signaling promoting microenvironment with low DKK1 that would support multiple pro-angiogenic signaling pathways (Saupe et al., 2013) (Figure 3).

In tenascin-C-deficient MEFs, reduced DKK2 levels were observed (Brellier et al., 2011a) suggesting that tenascin-C promotes DKK2 expression in fibroblasts. DKK1 and DKK2 have been shown to play opposite roles in angiogenesis; while DKK2 is promoting angiogenesis through stimulating filopodial dynamics and endothelial cell sprouting which involves LRP6-mediated APC/Asef2/Cdc42 activation, DKK1 has been shown to antagonize the pro-angiogenic DKK2 effect (Min et al., 2011), likely through competitive binding to LRP6. Since APC/Asef2/Cdc42 activation is LRP6 dependent and DKK1 sequesters LRP6 away from signaling complexes it will be important to determine whether the LRP6-mediated and DKK2 induced APC/Asef2/Cdc42 activation is blocked by DKK1 and potentially de-repressed by tenascin-C. It is possible that tenascin-C promotes tumor angiogenesis by altering the balance between the two DKK molecules, leading to low expression of DKK1 and high expression of DKK2. Since DKK1 and DKK2 are soluble factors they could exert a paracrine effect on surrounding endothelial and other cells.

Although tenascin-C is found in close proximity to tumor blood vessels there is no clear picture of whether and how a direct contact with tenascin-C promotes a pro-angiogenic behavior of endothelial cells. In addition to tumor blood vessels tenascin-C is also expressed in matrix tracks (reviewed in Midwood and Orend, 2009). This matrix network also expresses fibronectin, laminins, collagens and other extracellular matrix molecules. Most interestingly, in metastatic melanomas these tenascin-C tracks were described as lacking lymphatic and blood endothelial cells suggesting that they are not part of functional tumor vessels (Kaariainen et al., 2006). Instead of endothelial cells they contained erythrocytes and tumor cells which is suggestive of a connection to the vasculature. The absence of endothelial cells raises the question whether these tenascin-C matrix tracks once had been part of a vasculature before pruning had occurred. It remains to be seen what role tenascin-C plays in these networks. Given the presence of tumor cells within the tenascin-C matrix tracks may suggest that they potentially create a vasculature independent route for tumor cell dissemination (reviewed in Midwood and Orend, 2009).

In summary tenascin-C is functionally associated with tumor blood vessel formation (Figure 4). Tenascin-C may play multiple and even contradictory roles through its net-forming as well as its anti-adhesive activities in tumor angiogenesis which is still poorly understood and presumably context dependent. Tenascin-C promotes the angiogenic switch but does not promote the formation of productive tumor blood vessels. It is even possible that tenascin-C is involved in tumor vessel pruning. One important mechanism by which tenascin-C promotes tumor angiogenesis might involve downregulation of DKK1 thus creating a microenvironment prone to pro-angiogenic signaling. Given the pleiotrophic effects of DKK1 it is likely that other pro-angiogenic LRP6 dependent pathways (blocked by DKK1) are promoted (de-repressed) by tenascin-C due to DKK1 downregulation by tenascin-C. Given its prominent high expression in the tumor vasculature (and its large absence in healthy tissue) tenascin-C is an extraordinarily promising target in cancer therapy. This will be discussed in detail in Chapter 4.

## 2.4  Stem Cell Biology and Cell Plasticity

There is increasing evidence for the existence of tumor stem cell-like populations playing a role in tumor growth and metastasis (Reya et al., 2001). Several studies show that tenascin-C plays an important role in proliferation, migration, responsiveness to growth factors and differentiation of neural stem cells (NSC) or neural progenitors (Abaskharoun *et al.*, 2010; Czopka *et al.*, 2010; Garcion *et al.*, 2001; Garcion *et al.*, 2004; Moritz *et al.*, 2008; von Holst *et al.*, 2007; Yagi *et al.*, 2010). A number of recently published papers also investigated the role of tenascin-C in stemness of tumor cells such as in neuroblastoma (Pezzolo *et al.*, 2011), melanoma (Fukunaga-Kalabis *et al.*, 2010) and breast cancer (Oskarsson *et al.*, 2011).

### 2.4.1  Neural Stem Cells

Neural stem cells (NSC) are highly proliferative cells of neuronal origin, which are capable of self-renewal and differentiation into astrocytes, neurons or oligodendrocytes. Two studies examined the impact of tenascin-C knockout on neural stem cells in the central nervous system (CNS). Garcion and colleagues investigated the behaviour of oligodendrocyte progenitors (OP), which give rise to myelin-forming oligodendrocytes, in tenascin-C-null transgenic mice. OP cells of tenascin-C KO mice exhibited an increased migration along the optic nerve at P0 and P2. Those results were confirmed by *in vitro* experiments with rat OP and astroglial matrices derived from wild type or tenascin-C KO mice (Garcion *et al.*, 2001).

Tenascin-C-null mice also exhibited a decreased number of proliferative cells in the subventricular zone (SVZ). In this region OP cells are generated from pre-progenitor cells during early postnatal development. In addition double immunostaining for BrdU and the OP marker NG2 showed a reduction in proliferating OP cells in the CNS of tenascin-C KO mice. *In vitro* the authors demonstrated that tenascin-C regulated the proliferation of OP by sensitizing OP cells to the growth factor PDGF. OP cells from KO mice grown on tenascin-C-deficient astroglia matrix did not show any response to PDGF while wild type cells grown on a wild type matrix showed an optimal response. An antibody blocking β3 integrin inhibited the mitogenic effect of PDGF on rat OP cells in the presence of tenascin-C suggesting that tenascin-C might have a positive impact on the formation of a complex comprised of integrin αvβ3 and PDGFR (Schneller *et al.*, 1997).

Garcion and colleagues investigated in more detail the role of tenascin-C in regulating the responsiveness of neural stem cells to growth factors (Garcion *et al.*, 2004). Early embryonic neural stem cells respond to bFGF signaling only while late embryonic and adult neural stem cells by expressing EGFR do also respond to the mitogenic EGF stimulus (Qian *et al.*, 2000). By immunostaining the authors found delayed acquisition of

EGFR in tenascin-C knockout brain tissue of embryonic mice. *In vitro* the authors confirmed that neural stem cells derived from tenascin-C KO mice do not respond to EGF stimulation. In the presence of EGF neurospheres were obtained from telencephalic cells from E10.5 wild type mice while no neurospheres could be obtained from tenascin-C KO mice. In further support, tenascin-C-deficient cells isolated from E10.5 mice did not express EGFR in response to bFGF which stimulates the expression of EGFR while wild type cells did and, this defect could be rescued by addition of exogenous tenascin-C (Garcion *et al.*, 2004; Lillien and Raphael, 2000). Moreover the authors showed reduced proliferation in bFGF stimulated neural stem cells derived from E12.5 and P0 tenascin-C KO mice, indicating that tenascin-C enhances mitogenic bFGF signaling (Garcion *et al.*, 2004). In contrast to an enhanced EGFR expression in NSC by bFGF, BMP was shown to inhibit EGFR expression (Lillien and Raphael, 2000). Interestingly the inhibition of EGFR expression by BMP4 was only shown in neural stem cells derived from E12.5 and P0 tenascin-C KO mice but not in wild type mice, suggesting that tenascin-C also acts as an inhibitor of BMP4 signaling (Garcion *et al.*, 2004). In summary the authors have shown that tenascin-C modulates the responsiveness of neural stem cells to mitogenic stimuli by promoting the expression of EGFR, this is mediated by enhanced bFGF signaling as well as by inhibition of BMP4 signaling (Garcion *et al.*, 2004). Furthermore the authors showed that tenascin-C had an effect on the potential of NSC to differentiate into brain-forming cells (neurons, glial cells or oligodendrocytes). Although there was no change in the number of glial cells between wild type and KO mice, tenascin-C inhibited neurogenesis (Garcion *et al.*, 2004).

As tenascin-C has been described to undergo alternative splicing (see section 1.3) it is not surprising that also in NSC different tenascin-C isoforms were detected (von Holst *et al.*, 2007). By using primers flanking the alternatively spliced region of tenascin-C in RT-PCR analysis followed by dot blot hybridization analysis the expression of 20 tenascin-C isoforms in E13 neurospheres were shown. Tenascin-C isoforms contained up to 6 alternatively spliced TNIII domains. Addressing the underlying mechanism of alternative splicing of tenascin-C in NSC, the authors showed that the paired box transcription factor Pax6, a regulator of tenascin-C expression (Gotz *et al.*, 1998), enhances the expression of tenascin-C isoforms with more than three additional TNIII domains while the expression of isoforms with one or without any alternatively spliced TNIII domains was even decreased. Although Pax6 involvement could not explain the appearance of the seemingly NSC specific A1A4BD isoform, it was clearly shown that Pax6 differentially regulates alternative splicing of tenascin-C mRNA. Alternative splicing of tenascin-C by Pax6 seems to be restricted to NSC, as overexpression of Pax6 in MEF or in an astrocytic cell line did not alter tenascin-C isoform identity or abundance. Moritz and colleagues showed that tenascin-C reduced the expression of Sam68 in NSC (Moritz *et al.*, 2008). Sam68 is an RNA binding protein of the STAR family involved in mRNA splicing (Itoh *et al.*, 2002; Tremblay and Richard, 2006). Conversely, over expression of Sam68 in NSC grown as neurospheres was shown to promote the expression of large tenascin-C isoforms, suggesting that Sam68 regulates alternative splicing of tenascin-C (Moritz *et al.*, 2008).

Czopka and colleagues analysed in more detail the processes underlying tenascin-C induced retardation of OP differentiation into myelin basic protein (MBP)-positive oligodendrocytes. The authors demonstrated that tenascin-C bound to the cell adhesion molecule contactin and the Src family kinase Fyn, located in the lipid rafts of the OP membrane, diminished Akt phosphorylation and downstream inhibited expression of MBP and Sam68 (Czopka *et al.*, 2010).

Yagi and colleagues showed that tenascin-C expressed by NSC exhibits the human natural killer-1 (HNK-1) epitope on the cell surface. Similar to tenascin-C, HNK-1 is downregulated during the process of differentiation and facilitates the formation of neurospheres and enhances NSC proliferation. Furthermore the authors show that both tenascin-C and HNK-1 regulate the expression of EGFR in NSC which, given the demonstrated impact of tenascin-C on EGFR expression, suggests a potential interdependence of tenascin-C and HNK-1 in regulating EGFR expression (Yagi *et al.*, 2010). It remains to be seen whether HNK-1 is mediating this effect in a tenascin-C dependent manner.

Altogether, these studies demonstrated that tenascin-C modulates the responsiveness of neural stem cells to mitogenic stimuli and therefore enhances their proliferation. Furthermore, tenascin-C impacts on progenitor migration and differentiation of neural stem cells and progenitors.

## 2.4.2   Tumor Derived Endothelial Cells

Ricci-Vitiani *et al.* (2010) and Wang *et al.* (2010) first described that CD133+ glioblastoma stemlike cells are able to transdifferentiate into tumor-derived endothelial cells (TEC) and contribute to the formation of a tumor vasculature (Ricci-Vitiani *et al.*, 2010; Wang *et al.*, 2010b). Pezzolo and colleagues showed that tenascin-C contributes to the process of tumor stem cell transdifferentiation into TEC, which was demonstrated in neuroblastoma. Tenascin-C was mostly co-expressed with the neuroblastoma stem cell marker Oct4 in perivascular regions. This coexpression of tenascin-C and Oct4 was also seen in human neuroblastomas and in their orthotopic murine xenografts. Upon injection of cells not expressing tenascin-C orthotopic tumors lacked the lining of endothelial microvessels with TEC. In addition orthotopic tumors with expression of tenascin-C exhibited a higher microvessel density. *In vitro* the authors demonstrated the plasticity of tenascin-C expressing neuroblastoma cells where neuroblastoma cells were only able to grow as neurospheres if they expressed tenascin-C. Furthermore it was demonstrated that tenascin-C contributed to the differentiation into TEC by showing that tenascin-C expressing cells displayed an increased tube formation in matrigel. Upon culturing in VEGF-containing medium tenascin-C expressing cells acquired expression of endothelial-specific markers as PSMA, VE-Cadherin and CD31 while selected cells not expressing tenascin-C did not. Since in the applied FACS sorting approach it cannot be excluded that other molecules than tenascin-C are contributing to the described effect the published results await a confirmation by a tenascin-C knock down approach (Pezzolo *et al.*, 2011). Together these results suggest that tenascin-C is a characteristic marker of a stem cell microenvironment and could trigger stem cell proliferation. Moreover tenascin-C also plays a role in the plasticity of these cells contributing to their differentiation into TEC.

### 2.4.3 Cancer Stem Cells

Studies by Fukunaga-Kalabis and colleagues suggest that tenascin-C is a marker for stem cells in melanoma. By using oncosphere growth as readout for stemness the authors showed that tenascin-C is expressed in WM 3734 melanoma cells when they were grown as spheres but not when cultured in adherent conditions. It was demonstrated that tenascin-C is crucial for sphere growth of the melanoma cells since a tenascin-C knock down decreased sphere formation (Fukunaga-Kalabis *et al.*, 2010). In addition, tenascin-C knock down led to a decrease of the stem cell like side population expressing the ATP binding cassette transporter ABCB5. Expression of this transporter mediates the efflux capacity for the chemo-

therapeutic drug doxorubicin. Upon tenascin-C knock down the mela-
nomaspheres were significantly sensitized to doxorubicin. These results
suggest that tenascin-C expression in melanoma cells does not only contribute to the stemness phenotype but also promotes their drug resistance.

The study of Oskarsson and colleagues demonstrated that in metastatic breast cancer cells tenascin-C expression was important for the formation and fitness of oncospheres. Tenascin-C also had an impact on the
expression of the adult stem cell markers musashi homolog 1 (MSI1) and
LGR5, which are believed to be crucial for initiation of metastasis (Barker
*et al.*, 2007; Okano *et al.*, 2005). However tenascin-C was dispensable for
the expression of the pluripotency markers Nanog, Oct4 and Sox2. Furthermore tenascin-C did not affect the CD44+CD24- antigen profile,
which has been shown to be a characteristic marker for breast cancer stem
cells (Oskarsson *et al.*, 2011). Altogether these studies suggest that tenascin-C plays an important role in the stemness phenotype by supporting
recruitment, proliferation and plasticity of stem cells, progenitors and
cancer stem cells. It will be crucial to elucidate the downstream signaling
pathways regulated by tenascin-C, especially with the knowledge that
cancer stem cells seem to be instrumental for tumor growth and metastasis with the need for therapeutic approaches specifically targeting these
cells.

# Chapter 3

# The Role of Tenascin-C in Metastasis Formation

Metastasis occurs when tumor cells spread from the primary site and form a new tumor at a different site within the same or another organ. This process involves tumor cell migration, vessel invasion and extravasation into the distant organ tissue. While tumor cells travel in the blood or lymphatic circulation they need to survive. Only a few selected tumor cells that have gained the ability to leave the circulation and penetrate into the tissue of the secondary organ will grow into a new tumor (Chambers *et al.*, 2002).

## 3.1 Tenascin-C Promotes Metastasis Formation

Several studies showed that tenascin-C is not only a predictor for poor prognosis (see section 1.2) but in several cancers high tenascin-C expression also correlates with metastasis to distant organs such as lymph nodes, liver and lung (for an overview see Table 6). In contrast to these studies supporting a role of tenascin-C in metastasis there are also studies showing that tenascin-C expression does not correlate with metastasis or that a high tenascin-C expression exhibits an inverse correlation with metastasis (see Table 6). This discrepancy of the described studies might be due to the analysed patient material or differences in the protocol used for the disease assessment and there is clearly a need for further investigations.

Three studies from the same laboratory on a large cohort of human breast cancer specimen support the possibility that tenascin-C may be a predictor for lung metastasis (Minn *et al.*, 2005; Oskarsson *et al.*, 2011; Tavazoie *et al.*, 2008). A metastasis promoting impact of tenascin-C in breast cancer was demonstrated in murine xenograft experiments.

| Organ | Tenascin-C correlation with metastasis and/or invasion | References |
|---|---|---|
| | **Breast** | |
| Small node-negative carcinoma | Staining at the invasion border but general stromal staining is no predictor for metastasis | (Jahkola et al., 1996) |
| Intraductal carcinoma | Stromal staining correlates with early invasion | (Jahkola et al., 1998a) |
| Axillary node-negative carcinoma | Expression at invasion boarder serves as prognostic factor for local recurrence | (Jahkola et al., 1998b) |
| Breast carcinoma | Positivity in cancer cells and stroma correlates with lymph node metastasis | (Ishihara et al., 1995) |
| Invasive breast carcinoma | No correlation with lymph node metastasis | (Shoji et al., 1993) |
| Benign tumors and ductal and lobular carcinoma | Increased expression and stromal staining in infiltrating carcinomas | (Gould et al., 1990) |
| Carcinoma | Changes in expression during menstrual cycle; increased stromal staining of infiltrating carcinomas | (Ferguson et al., 1990) |
| Primary invasive breast carcinoma | Tenascin-C expression at the invasive front was positively correlated with lymph node status | (Ioachim et al., 2002) |
| Infiltrating ductal carcinoma | Expression of tenascin-C in tumors with lymph node metastasis is higher than in those without lymph node metastasis | (Wang et al., 2010a) |
| Primary breast cancer | Tenascin-C mRNA expression no correlation with nodal status, tenascin-C was significantly associated with metastasis free survival of adjuvant tamoxifen-treated patients | (Helleman et al., 2008) |
| Breast cancer | Tenascin-C expression in primary tumor and lung metastatic foci is associated with lung metastatic relapse. | (Oskarsson et al., 2011) |

| | Kidney | |
|---|---|---|
| Bladder neoplasia | Strong staining in stroma of invasive tumors | (Deen and Ball, 1994) |
| Inflammation and neoplasm of urinary bladder | Increased staining with inflammation and more intense in transitional cell carcinomas with strong stromal staining in infiltrating carcinoma cells | (Tiitta et al., 1993) |
| Clear cell renal cell carcinoma | Tenascin-C expression was an independent predictor of metastasis in patients with stage 1-3 disease. | (Ohno et al., 2008) |
| | Lung | |
| Cancers with variety of clinicopathological features | Large tenascin-C isoforms found in cancer tissue and tenascin-C degradation is a marker for the metastatic potential | (Kusagawa et al., 1998) |
| Mesothelioma | Staining of malignant tumors at invasive front | (Procopio et al., 1998) |
| Non-small cell lung cancer | Tenascin-C expression was frequently observed in tumors with LN metastasis (P =0.06) | (Han et al., 2003) |
| | Female genital tract and ovaries | |
| Endometrial carcinoma | Tenascin-C correlates with metastasis, muscle and vascular invasion | (Doi et al., 1996) |
| | Salivary glands | |
| Hyalinizing clear cell carcinoma of the salivary gland | Stromal marker for invasive front | (Felix et al., 2002) |
| Salivary gland tumors | Is higher in carcinomas ex-pleomorphic adenomas than in pleomorphic adenomas and correlates with disease progression (metastasis) | (Felix et al., 2004) |
| | Other glands | |
| Pancreatic carcinoma | Identification of invasion promoting stroma | (Linder et al., 2001) |
| Pancreatic carcinoma | Is increased in carcinomas but does not correlate with poor differentiation, decreased survival, clinical stage or metastasis | (Juuti et al., 2004) |
| Insulinoma | Is increased in insulinomas with lymph node or liver metastasis | (Saupe et al., 2013) |
| Pancreatic adenocarcinoma | Fibrilliar tenascin-C expression is associated with liver metastasis | (Chen et al., 2009) |

| Gastro-intestinal tract | | |
|---|---|---|
| Gastric carcinoma | Strong stromal staining correlates with low stage but not with nodal status or metastasis | (Wiksten et al., 2003) |
| Colitis, colon adenoma and colorectal carcinoma | No BM staining at bottom of crypts in normal tissue, loss of this polarity in colitis, increased stromal staining in adenomas and carcinomas; correlation with lymph node metastasis | (Riedl et al., 1992) |
| Adenoma and carcinoma | Correlation between transcript levels and depth of invasion and frequency of metastasis to lymph nodes | (Hanamura et al., 1997) |
| Gastric carcinoma | No correlation with invasion, metastasis, survival | (Ilunga and Iriyama, 1995) |
| Gastric carcinoma and lymph node metastasis | No correlation with invasion, metastasis or prognosis | (Ikeda et al., 1995) |
| Colonic carcinoma with and without lymphogeneous metastasis | Very strong expression in every non-metastatic case; good correlation with prognosis | (Sugawara et al., 1991) |
| Colorectal cancer | Tenascin-C expression in tumor invasive area was significantly correlated with tumor progression, lymphatic invasion, lymph node metastasis and advanced pTNM stage | (Ide et al., 2007) |
| Gastric adenocarcinoma, colorectal adenocarcinoma, gastric adjacent non-cancerous mucosa and colorectal adjacent non-cancerous mucosa | Tenascin-C expression was negatively correlated with liver metastasis, but not with depth of invasion, venous invasion or lymph node metastasis. | (Zheng et al., 2007) |
| Diffuse and intestinal type gastric carcinoma | Enhanced staining in the stroma of invasive tumors | (Tiitta et al., 1994b) |

| Head and neck | | |
|---|---|---|
| Oral squamous cell carcinoma | High transcript levels correlate with lymph node metastasis | (Nagata et al., 2003) |
| Oral tongue squamous cell carcinoma | Tenascin-C mRNA expression showed no statistical significance both in negative and in positive lymph node metastasis patients although a trend was observed. Tenascin-C is a prognostic factor for survival. | (Wang et al., 2010b) |
| Squamous carcinoma of the floor of the mouth | Marker for *in situ* and invasive squamous carcinoma | (Regezi et al., 2002) |
| Laryngeal squamous cell carcinoma, dysplasias, papilloma | Stromal staining correlates with malignancy but not the histological grade of invasive carcinomas | (Goussia et al., 2000) |
| Laryngeal squamous carcinoma | Strong staining in invasive carcinomas | (Hagedorn et al., 1999) |
| Laryngeal carcinoma | stromal marker around cancer nests, cytoplasmic staining of cancer cells in majority of invasive carcinomas | (Yoshida et al., 1999) |
| Laryngeal squamous carcinoma | Stromal marker of carcinoma *in situ* and invasive carcinomas | (Uhlman and Niehans, 1999) |
| Oral squamous carcinoma | Intracellular tenascin-C staining in cancer cells of the invasive front | (Mori et al., 1996) |
| Oral squamous cell carcinoma | Enhanced stromal expression in invasive tumors with strongest expression at advancing edges of tumors | (Tiitta et al., 1994a) |
| Leukoplakia and oral squamous cell carcinoma | Increase in submucosa correlating with degree of hyperplasia/dysplasia and more intense and extending into stroma in SCC at the infiltrating tumor margin | (Shrestha et al., 1994) |
| Skin | | |
| Melanoma | Higher expression in lesions of greater dermal invasiveness | (Natali et al., 1990) |
| Merkel cell carcinoma | Tenascin-C expression increased with tumor size and malignancy at sites of invasive growth, no correlation with metastasis | (Koljonen et al., 2005) |

| | | |
|---|---|---|
| Primary melanoma | Absence of tenascin-C in stroma at invasion front correlates with lower risk for metastasis | (Ilmonen et al., 2004) |
| Extramammary Paget's disease | No correlation with level of invasion | (Kuivanen et al., 2004) |
| benign, dysplastic and malignant melanocytic tumors | Correlation with malignancy and metastasis | (Tuominen and Kallioinen, 1994) |
| Primary melanomas | Intensity of tenascin-C staining correlated with incidence of sentinel node micrometastases. | (Kaariainen et al., 2006) |
| Skeleton and teeth | | |
| Odontogenic tumors | Staining at epithelial-mesenchymal interfaces in ameloblastomas and adenomatoid tumors and widespread stromal staining in fibromas and odontomas | (Mori et al., 1995) |
| Osteosarcoma | Correlation with metastasis and poor survival | (Tanaka et al., 2000) |
| Primary giant cell tumors | Tenascin-C expression (microarray) correlates with metastasis | (Pazzaglia et al., 2010) |
| Soft tissues, lymphomas | | |
| Pediatric rhabdomyosarcoma | All tumors stain positive without correlation to tumor differentiation or metastasis | (Saxon et al., 1997) |
| Prostate | | |
| Prostatic adenocarcinoma | Expression of large splice variants by carcinoma cells at tumor invasion front | (Katenkamp et al., 2004) |

**Table 6:** Correlation of tenascin-C expression in cancer with invasion and metastasis. These data are adapted from supplementary Table 1 in Orend and Chiquet-Ehrismann (2006) and completed with new studies.

By tail vein injection of human MDAMB-231 cells into immune compromised nude mice tumor cells were selected that homed to the lung. Upon transcriptomic microarray analysis on the highly lung metastatic versus the low lung metastatic cell line tenascin-C was identified in a gene signature that correlated with lung metastasis (Minn *et al.*, 2005; Tavazoie *et al.*, 2008). Calvo *et al.* (2008) used another xenograft model, where tenascin-C MDAMB 435 cells lacking TNC expression upon knock down were injected into the mammary fat pad of nude mice. Also in this model a lowered tenascin-C expression correlated with a reduced lung metastasis (Calvo *et al.*, 2008). Calvo and colleagues observed tenascin-C to be increased in MMTV-Myc induced breast tumors overexpressing VEGF that gave rise to micro- and macrometastasis which was in contrast to mice not overexpressing VEGFA where tenascin-C expression and the metastasis rate were low. By comparison of the genes upregulated in the MMTV-Myc/VEGF tumors and upon comparison to genes upregulated in human breast cancer with metastasis, tenascin-C again turned out as a candidate of a lung specific metastasis signature (Calvo *et al.*, 2008).

In contrast to these studies with a positive link of tenascin-C to lung metastasis in breast cancer, in two other studies no correlation of tenascin-C expression and metastasis was observed. Ramaswamy and colleagues compared the gene expression profile of adenocarcinoma derived metastasis of multiple tumors including breast cancer to unmatched primary adenocarcinomas (Ramaswamy *et al.*, 2003). Landemaine and colleagues compared the gene expression signature from lung breast cancer derived metastasis with that of other non-pulmonary sites (Landemaine *et al.*, 2008). This not understood discrepancy warrants further investigation.

There is evidence that tenascin-C plays also a role in bone metastasis (Oskarsson *et al.*, 2011). The authors showed that upon knock down of tenascin-C in breast cancer cell line MDAMB231 (selected to home to the lung, bone and brain) less metastasis was observed in the lung and bones but not the liver nor brain. However, it needs to be determined why and how tenascin-C specifically influences the seeding, survival or proliferation of metastasis-initiating cells in certain organs while at other sites tenascin-C does not seem to play a role. It is possible that other extracellular matrix molecules or microenvironmental factors contribute to this site specific seeding of cancer cells, which may occur in conjunction with or independently of tenascin-C.

Since tenascin-C has been shown to have immuno-modulatory functions (see section 2.2) the presented data might be hampered by the fact that the studies have been done in immuno-deficient mice. Also the stromal compartment in a murine host is different from that of the human tumor (Fantozzi and Christofori, 2006) and, human cells are not fully adapted to grow in a murine environment (Kuperwasser et al., 2005). In this context the studies by O'Connell et al. (2011) and Saupe et al. (2013) are important. O'Connell and colleagues have used the 4T1 Balb/c grafting model. Upon intravenous injection of syngeneic 4T1 cells into an immune competent tenascin-C KO host less metastatic lesions were observed in the lung (O'Connell et al., 2011). Curiously, metastasis assessment was only documented 4 days after intravenous 4T1 cell engraftment. Whether at later time points the absence of tenascin-C in the stroma had an impact on metastasis was not mentioned. It was also not addressed whether the complete and simultaneous absence of tenascin-C from the tumor cells and the host had an impact on metastasis.

This latter question had been addressed in the PNET/Rip1Tag2 model. Although these mice (in particular in a C57Bl6 background) are not the most appropriate model to address metastasis because mice die due to hypoglycemia before they can develop macrometastasis, a recent publication demonstrated that the expression levels of tenascin-C had an impact on micrometastasis formation in this immune competent and genetic model of stochastic tumorigenesis (Saupe et al., 2013). The authors had assessed micrometastasis formation by tissue staining and qRT-PCR for insulin in liver and lung tissue. No macrometastases were seen. Also, in liver tissue no difference in micrometastasis was seen irrespective of the tenascin-C copy number, yet differences in insulin expression levels were noted in lung tissue. Whereas the lowest insulin levels were seen in tenascin-C null tumor mice, insulin expression was highest in lungs from tumor mice with expression of transgenic tenascin-C. The qRT-PCR results were confirmed qualitatively by tissue staining and showed insulin expression within the lung parenchyma, thus suggesting that the insulin signal derived from lesions in the lung rather than from circulating tumor cells (Saupe et al., 2013). Although the result was anticipated, this is the first study where in an immune competent context with stochastic tumor and metastasis formation an impact of tenascin-C on metastasis has been proven.

In contrast to the presented studies Talts and colleagues had used another genetic model with stochastic breast tumor development and lung metastasis. Tenascin-C null mice were crossed with MMTV/PyMT (poly-omavirus (PyV) middle T oncogene under the transcriptional control of the mouse mammary tumor virus (MMTV) long-terminal repeat) transgenic mice, which spontaneously develop adenocarcinomas in the mammary gland that metastasize to the lung. In this model the authors observed neither a difference in tumor growth and size nor in the number of metastasis in the lung (Talts *et al.*, 1999). But organization of the tumor nests and extracellular matrix was different and the tumors were more infiltrated by macrophages in the absence of tenascin-C. These data suggest that other mechanisms may have promoted lung metastasis in the absence of tenascin-C. What these mechanisms are and whether they are a direct consequence of the absence of tenascin-C remains to be seen.

Not only does the overall expression of tenascin-C in the primary tumor seem to be important for a higher risk of metastasis but also its organization, the source and the place of expression. Chen and colleagues showed that only the fibrillar organization of tenascin-C in pancreatic cancer correlated with metastasis. As MMP2 expression correlated with fibrilliar tenascin-C, the authors suggested that for the fibrilliar organization of tenascin-C the presence of MMP2 is required. Indeed in *in vitro* experiments co-culture of stromal fibroblasts with metastatic pancreatic cancer cells triggered fibrilliar tenascin-C organization, and most importantly this was suppressed by an MMP2 inhibitor (Chen *et al.*, 2009). Moreover, non-metastatic pancreatic cancer cells deposited fibrilliar tenascin-C only upon addition of exogenous MMP2. A concomitant high expression of MMP2 and tenascin-C in the identified gene signature for breast cancer lung metastasis (Calvo *et al.*, 2008) seems to support a potential link of tenascin-C and MMP2 to metastasis. Future studies need to address how MMP2 is linked to fibrillar tenascin-C and whether and how MMP2 affects tenascin-C organization into fibrillar tenascin-C matrix tracks that at least in melanoma have been clearly demonstrated to correlate with metastasis formation (Kaariainen *et al.*, 2006).

Several studies showed that not the overall expression of tenascin-C in the tumor is important but that the expression of tenascin-C at the tumor invasion front correlates with metastasis. This has been shown in colorectal carcinoma (Ide *et al.*, 2007), primary invasive breast carcinoma (Ioachim *et al.*, 2002; Oskarsson *et al.*, 2011), early breast cancer and axillary node-negative breast carcinoma (Jahkola *et al.*, 1998a; Jahkola *et al.*, 1998b; Jahkola *et al.*, 1996). These results suggest a role for tenascin-C in epithelial mesenchymal transition (EMT), cancer cell migration and inva-

sion, processes which have been demonstrated to be fundamental for metastasis formation (see next section).

In summary there is increasing evidence that in several cancers tenascin-C promotes metastasis. The correlation of high tenascin-C expression
in the primary tumor to the formation of lung metastasis is demonstrated
in several immunohistochemical and gene expression analysis-based
studies and has been recapitulated in a few murine tumor models. To
address the underlying mechanism and to gain useful knowledge for
human cancer diagnosis and therapy, better murine cancer metastasis
models with an intact immune system and stochastic tumorigenesis are
needed.

## 3.2    Tenascin-C Promotes Cancer Cell Migration, Invasion and EMT

In several *in vitro* models with a variety of tumor cells (breast, colon cancer, glioma, chondrosarcoma, squamous cell carcinoma) tenascin-C has
been demonstrated to increase migration and invasion (Table 7). A particular role of tenascin-C was demonstrated by a tenascin-C knock down
approach. Tumors derived from GBM cells knocked down for tenascin-C
and engrafted into nude mice consisted of less infiltrating
tumor cells and less tumor cell clusters in the surrounding brain tissue,
despite the fact that no difference in tumor growth and proliferation was
observed (Hirata *et al.*, 2009).

Tenascin-C also appears to play a role in the intricate cross talk of
myofibroblasts with tumor cells. Myofibroblasts isolated from colon cancer tissue stimulated the invasive behaviour of colon cancer cells in a
tenascin-C dependent manner (De Wever *et al.*, 2004). Colon cancer cells
co-cultured with myofibroblasts rapidly invaded a collagen gel which
could be blocked by treatment with an antibody against the tenascin-C
EGFR repeats, suggesting that deposition of tenascin-C by the myofibroblasts in the gel drives the invasion of the cancer cells. The authors linked
this tenascin-C stimulated pro-invasive behaviour of carcinoma cells to
down regulation of RhoA signaling (De Wever *et al.*, 2004). Similarly,
Gaggioli and colleagues observed that squamous carcinoma cells invade
an organotypic matrix upon co-culture with stromal fibroblasts that were
derived from oral or vulval squamous cell carcinoma. Stromal fibroblasts
invaded and strongly modified the matrix by promoting degradation and
deposition of matrix including tenascin-C and fibronectin. The collagen

| Cell line | TNC | Assay | Reference |
|---|---|---|---|
| | | Breast cancer | |
| Mouse cancer cell line, GHOM5E, was established from a spontaneously developing tumor in a congenic TNC-null mouse of the GRS/A strain | TNC (3 µg/ml) added to the medium | Transwell migration assay — increased migration compared to no treatment | (Tsunoda et al., 2003) |
| MDAMB 231 | Added to the medium (10 µg/ml) | Matrigel invasion assay - Cells were plated on inserts pre-coated or untreated with Matrigel, 6h — stimulates invasion together with TGFβ1 | (Ilunga et al., 2004) |
| LM2 (derived from MDAMB 231, selected to metastasize to the lung, details in (Minn et al., 2005) | TNC knock down | Transwell invasion — decreased invasion compared to CTR SH | (Tavazoie et al., 2008) |
| M630 (Cell line from a Myc/VEGF tumor) | TNC blocking antibody | Wound closure — decreased migration compared to control, IgG treatment did not affect migration | (Calvo et al., 2008) |
| MDAMB 435 | TNC knock down | Wound closure — decreased migration compared to CTR SH | (Calvo et al., 2008) |
| MDAMB 231, MCF-7, T47D, MDDAMB 468 | Overexpression of TNC isoforms with TNIII D or TNIII BD domains | Tumor cell invasion in real time with modified Boyden Chamber Assay — increased invasion compared to empty vector control | (Hancox et al., 2009) |

| Cell line | Treatment | Assay | Result | Reference |
|---|---|---|---|---|
| MCF-7, T47D | Overexpression of the TNC isoform containing TNIII BAD1D domains | Tumor cell invasion in real time with modified Boyden Chamber Assay, up to 48 hrs | increased invasion compared to empty vector control | (Guttery et al., 2010b) |
| MCF-7 | adding 10 µg/ml TNC to the medium | Wound healing | increased migration | (Nagaharu et al., 2011) |
| MD AMB231-LM2 (Minn et al., 2005) | TNC knock down | Matrigel invasion/Transwell membrane | decreased invasion compared to SH CTR | (Oskarsson et al., 2011) |
| Brain tumor | | | | |
| U251.3 | TNC coating (20 µg/ml) | Coating of undersurface of transwell membranes, 4 hrs | increased migration compared to FN or BSA | (Deryugina & Bourdon, 1996) |
| U251.3 | TNC coating (10 µg/ml) | Spheroid outgrowth assay, 1 or 2 days | increased migration compared to FN | (Deryugina & Bourdon, 1996) |
| U178, U251 | 10 µg/ml embedded in the matrix | 3D collagen I matrix, transwell invasion chamber | increased invasion | (Sarkar et al., 2006) |
| LN229 | TNC knock down | Wound healing assay, 14h | decreased migration | (Hirata et al., 2009) |
| LN229 | TNC knock down | Single cell locomotion assay, 12h | decreased migration, reversed by coating with 10 µg/ml TNC | (Hirata et al., 2009) |

| WM35, WM983, WM983B | Single cell tracking | TNC coating (2µg/cm²) together with collagen | increased speed but no difference for displacement/track length) compared to collagen coating alone | (Grahovac et al., 2012) |
|---|---|---|---|---|
| **Colon cancer** | | | | |
| HCT-8/E11, PC/AA/C1 | Invasion of cells seeded on top of collagen gel, 24h | Blocking TNC with BC24 antibody | decreased invasion compared to IgG treatment | (De Wever et al., 2004) |
| HCT-8/E11 | Invasion of cells seeded on top of collagen I, 24h | TNC (soluble or matrix-embedded – 1 or 2 µg/ml) | increased invasiveness together with SF/HGF | (De Wever et al., 2004) |
| **Squamous cell carcinoma** | | | | |
| SCC12 | Cells seeded on organotypic matrix enriched with CAF | siRNA mediated knock down in CAF | no effect | (Gaggioli et al., 2007) |
| **Bone cancer** | | | | |
| JJ012 chondrosarcoma | Collagen based cell invasion assay | TNC coating (10 µg/ml) | increased invasion compared to FN or BSA | (Galoian et al., 2007) |

**Table 7:** Tenascin-C modulates tumor cell migration and invasion *in vitro*.

matrix within these tracks was organized into thick bundles (Gaggioli *et al.*, 2007). The authors demonstrated that those tracks promoted carcinoma cell invasion. However, tenascin-C and fibronectin seemed not to be crucial for the invasion, as a knock down of both molecules in fibroblasts did not change the number of invading carcinoma cells. What the role of tenascin-C in this context is remained elusive.

It is conceivable that the fibrillar tenascin-C matrix observed in pancreatic cancer (Chen *et al.*, 2009) and in melanoma (Kaariainen *et al.*, 2006) has similarities with the tenascin-C matrix tracks observed in cell culture (Gaggioli *et al.*, 2007). Kaariainen and colleagues showed that in melanoma where tenascin-C mRNA expression correlated with invasiveness and metastatic lesions, tenascin-C is assembled together with several other extracellular matrix molecules such as fibronectin, laminins and procollagen I within channels or matrix tracks. It was shown that melanoma cells are located within these matrix channels which supports a potential contribution of these channels to melanoma dissemination and metastasis (Kaariainen *et al.*, 2006). Also other studies revealed a high expression of several matrix molecules (laminin-5 and collagens) together with tenascin-C in metastatic conditions, as shown in MMTV-VEGF/c-myc transgenic tumors compared to non-metastatic c-myc tumors (Calvo *et al.*, 2008). It is conceivable that a combined high expression of several extracellular matrix molecules and their assembly into matrix tracks or channels contributes to metastasis by e.g. providing dissemination cues and/or local niches that promote survival of disseminated tumor cells. The role of tenascin-C expression in matrix tracks has been furthermore extensively addressed in these two reviews (Midwood *et al.*, 2011; Van Obberghen-Schilling *et al.*, 2011a).

However it is unknown what the exact role of tenascin-C within these matrix channels would be, as could be envisaged promotion of survival, proliferation and/or migration of tumor and tumor associated cells. A potential supportive role is not unlikely given the organization of tenascin-C in matrix tracks and its promoting effect on survival (Oskarsson *et al.*, 2011, Saupe et al 2013), proliferation (Huang *et al.*, 2001; Orend and Chiquet-Ehrismann, 2006) and migration of tumor cells (see **Table 7**). Another question is whether and how these tenascin-C matrix channels play a role in tumor cell dissemination throughout the entire body. These matrix channels were not lined by blood nor lymphatic endothelial cells (excluding that they are a physical component of functional vessels) but exhibited erythrocytes which supports a connection of the tumor mass to the circulation through the tenascin-C matrix channels. Yet, mechanistic proof is missing that would provide an active involvement of these matrix channels in tumor cell dissemination and metastasis. Moreover, it is unknown whether tenascin-C plays a role in the formation and/or function of these matrix channels.

Grahovac and colleagues showed that the EGFL repeats of tenascin-C in particular might regulate migration and invasion of melanoma cells. Overexpression of the tenascin-C EGF-like domain in melanoma cells increased their invasion into matrigel (Grahovac et al., 2012). This could be blocked by a Rho-associated protein kinase (ROCK)-inhibitor, suggesting the involvement of a tenascin-C EGF-like induced cytoskeletal alteration in the process of matrigel invasion. However in 2D assays over expression of tenascin-C EGF-like rather decreased cell migration suggesting that the 3D organization of tenascin-C EGF-like domains is instrumental. These observations also raise the possibility that specific domains in tenascin-C might induce different cell responses. An over representation of specific tenascin-C domains mostly encompassing the alternatively spliced TNIII repeats but not the EGF-like repeats had been demonstrated in several cancers. In particular in breast cancer the expression of tenascin-C isoforms, containing TNIII D, TNIII BD or TNIII BAD1D domains, were associated with increased tumor cell invasion (Adams et al., 2002; Guttery et al., 2010b; Hancox et al., 2009). Exposure of certain domains within tenascin-C could also arise from cleavage of the molecule by MMPs and other proteases (reviewed in Midwood and Orend, 2009).

Tenascin-C itself might also increase the expression and activity of MMPs stimulating the invasive behaviour of cancer cells. Ilunga and colleagues showed that MDAMB231 invasion into matrigel was stimulated by the addition of both tenascin-C and TGFβ1, which could be blocked by a MMP-inhibitor (Ilunga et al., 2004). Similarly, tenascin-C also stimulated the invasion of glioblastoma cells by increasing protein kinase C δ activity and MMP12 expression and migration could be inhibited by MMP-inhibitors or an antibody specific for MMP12 (Sarkar et al., 2006; Sarkar and Yong, 2010).

EMT, characterized by the loss of epithelial cell-cell contacts and a gain of a fibroblast-like motile phenotype that enables tumor cell migration and invasion (Huber et al., 2005) is considered as a key process of tumor epithelial cells toward metastasis. There is evidence that EMT is promoting metastasis and that EMT often occurs at the invasive front of a tumor, where tenascin-C has been shown to be highly expressed (see Table 6). These frequent observations support a potential active role of tenascin-C in EMT.

In support of this possibility, in breast carcinoma tenascin-C expression correlated with the expression of the mesenchymal marker vimentin and, in several cancer cell lines tenascin-C and vimentin were found to be coexpressed (Dandachi *et al.*, 2001). Moreover, tenascin-C is highly expressed at the invasive front of colorectal tumors at sites with nuclear β-catenin (Beiter *et al.*, 2005). Nuclear β-catenin has been demonstrated to be an EMT marker (Kim *et al.*, 2002). Knock down of β-catenin in colon cancer cell lines indeed resulted in reduced tenascin-C expression and the authors provided evidence that β-catenin is directly regulating tenascin-C promoter activity (Beiter *et al.*, 2005) which suggests a positive feedback regulation. Nagaharu and colleagues demonstrated that upon a combined treatment with tenascin-C and TGFβ1 two breast cancer cell lines (MCF7 and T47-D) acquire an EMT-like phenotype, characterized by loss of membranous E-cadherin and β-catenin, which was linked to increased cell migration (Nagaharu *et al.*, 2011). A recent publication from the same group (Katoh *et al.*, 2013) demonstrates that tenascin-C binding to integrins αvβ1 and αvβ6 is an essential mechanism for the induction of EMT. The authors show that the integrin subunits αv, β1 and β6 bind to tenascin-C and that a combined treatment with tenascin-C and TGFβ1 markedly increased the expression of the integrin-subunit αv and β6. Furthermore integrin β6 and αv colocalized in focal adhesions and an increased heterodimerization of αv and β1 in focal adhesions upon tenascin-C treatment was observed. Importantly, tenascin-C-induced EMT was inhibited upon treatment with αv- and β1-blocking antibodies while tenascin-C/TGFβ1–induced EMT could be only inhibited by an αv-blocking antibody or combined treatment of αvβ6- and β1-blocking antibodies.

Furthermore tenascin-C seemed to be involved in regulating the EMT process in the mouse lens epithelium upon injury (Tanaka *et al.*, 2010). In another study tenascin-C promoted a partial EMT in MCF7 breast cancer cells that changed their cobblestone epithelial morphology into a fibroblastoid phenotype upon growth on a tenascin-C substratum. This was linked to an altered expression of the adaptor protein 14.3.3tau (Martin *et al.*, 2003).

These observations suggest that tenascin-C promotes EMT but may also be regulated by EMT, as it was shown to be a β-catenin target gene. Thus highly expressed tenascin-C at the tumor invasion front will enhance cancer cell migration and invasion. In summary, tenascin-C might increase cancer cell invasion and migration by promoting EMT and/or by enhancing the activity or expression of MMPs. Organisation of tenascin-C into fibrillar tenascin-C channels presumably plays another important role in metastasis (Figure 4).

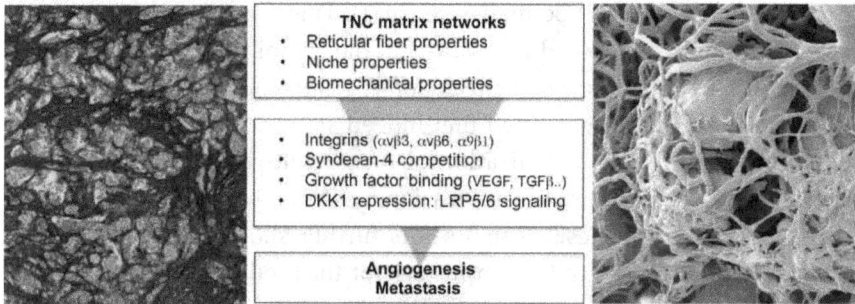

**Figure 4:** Tenascin-C niches in tumor tissue and impact on angiogenesis and metastasis. Pictures taken from Saupe et al., (2013). Left: Tenascin-C expression in a malignant human insulinoma. Right: scanning electron micrograph of the highly aberrant vasculature in a RT2/TNC insulinoma with transgenic tenascin-C expression.

## 3.3    Tenascin-C in the Metastatic Niche

Disseminated tumor cells which form metastasis in the tissue of a secondary organ need a perceptive microenvironment or niche that promotes survival and expansion at the secondary site. The seed and soil hypothesis argues that this niche can either be prepared by the arriving tumor cells (the seed) or by the organ microenvironment (the soil) that is already modulated by soluble factors secreted from cells of the primary tumor (Paget, 1989). The metastatic niche therefore is described as a specialized microenvironment which supports maintenance and growth of metastasis-initiating cells (Psaila and Lyden, 2009). Fibronectin and MMPs in the (pre-)metastatic niche seem to enable the seeding and survival of arriving metastatic cells (Psaila and Lyden, 2009). Given the involvement of tenascin-C in the primary tumor and in metastasis it is possible that tenascin-C plays a role both in the pre-metastatic and metastatic niche (schematically depicted in Figure 4).

Two recent studies addressed whether tenascin-C plays a role in preparing the metastatic niche. O'Connell and colleagues demonstrated that

S100A4 (Mts1/FSP) positive stromal cells, which are mesenchymal cells including fibroblasts are a source for tenascin-C. S100A4+ cells significantly contributed to metastasis in the lung upon injection of 4T1 breast cancer cells into a syngeneic host, since ablation of S100A4+ cells decreased the number of metastatic lesions in the lung. Moreover tenascin-C expression in the metastatic lung tissue was strongly reduced upon ablation of S100A4+ cells (O'Connell *et al.*, 2011). This argued for an important role of stromally expressed tenascin-C in the colonization and outgrowth of tumor cells in the lung. By means of 4T1 cells injected into tenascin-C KO mice the authors confirmed that indeed stromally provided tenascin-C is important for the colonization of tumor cells at the metastatic site. However a lack of tenascin-C expression by stromal cells did not induce a difference in angiogenesis. The authors further showed that VEGFA secreted by the S100A4+ cells is important for the seeding of the tumor cells in the lung (O'Connell *et al.*, 2011). Whether VEGFA plays a role in the preparation of a pro-angiogenic microenvironment as claimed by the authors or whether VEGFA supports survival (Lichtenberger *et al.*, 2010) is an open question. Together these results suggested that tenascin-C secreted by S100A4+ stromal cells promotes lung metastasis by preparation of a permissive microenvironment.

Oskarsson and colleagues demonstrated that tenascin-C provided by disseminated breast cancer cells plays an important role for the survival and growth of metastasis-initiating cells in the lung (Oskarsson *et al.*, 2011). However, expression of tenascin-C by the cancer cells itself seemed only to be crucial at early time points of the metastatic outgrowth while later knock down of tenascin-C did not affect growth of the metastatic lesions. This might be due to the fact that metastatic cells have already activated the surrounding stroma to express tenascin-C, most likely involving the S100A4+ cells identified by O'Connell *et al.* (2011). The authors further elucidated by which mechanism tenascin-C regulated the lung metastasis potential of breast cancer cells (Oskarsson *et al.*, 2011). Tenascin-C decreased apoptosis of cells in the metastasis site while it did not change their proliferation. Tenascin-C knock down in breast cancer oncospheres showed that tenascin-C indeed specifically promoted the survival of metastasis-initiating cells but not their self-renewal capacity. In this model tenascin-C expression was significantly enhanced in comparison to monolayer cultures and correlated with the expression of the pluripotency markers Sox2, Oct4 and Nanog and the adult stem cell markers MSI1 and LGR5. However, tenascin-C knock down revealed that tenascin-C is not regulating the expression of these putative pluripotency markers, while the activity of Wnt and Notch signaling was shown to be reduced in a tenascin-C dependent manner (Oskarsson et al., 2011). Using knock down and blocking strategies the authors concluded that tenascin-C regulates lung metastasis by stimulating the expression of the Wnt target LGR5 and suppressing JAK2-STAT5 signaling which would result in MSI1 induction and Notch pathway activation.

Other important extracellular matrix components playing a role in tumor progression and formation of metastasis have been shown to be co-expressed with tenascin-C and even bind to tenascin-C. In particular fibronectin and periostin have been shown to interact with tenascin-C. Interactions between fibronectin and tenascin-C were extensively reviewed (Van Obberghen-Schilling et al., 2011b). Kii and colleagues demonstrated that periostin is important for the incorporation of tenascin-C into the matrix meshwork probably due to bridging binding of tenascin-C to other extracellular matrix components such as fibronectin (Kii et al., 2010) although tenascin-C can also directly bind to fibronectin (Huang et al., 2001). Recently, Malanchi and colleagues demonstrated an important role for periostin in lung metastasis derived from breast cancer. The authors demonstrated Wnt ligand binding to periostin which seems to stimulate the colonization of metastasis-initiating cells (Malanchi et al., 2011). It is interesting to speculate that tenascin-C and periostin act together to promote the survival of metastasis initiating cells (Oskarsson and Massague, 2012); while periostin presents Wnt ligands to the cancer cells (Malanchi et al., 2011), tenascin-C downregulates the Wnt inhibitor DKK1 (Ruiz et al., 2004; Saupe et al., 2013), stabilizes β-catenin (Ruiz et al., 2004) and promotes expression of the Wnt target genes LGR5 (Oskarsson et al., 2011), Axin2, CD44, cyclin D1 and Slug (Saupe et al., 2013).

In malignant cancers tenascin-C is found assembled into networks/tracks that may originate from an inappropriately turned on reticular fiber program that would create fibrillar tube like tenascin-C networks (together with other extracellular matrix molecules) in thymus and spleen, where it is believed that these structures provide guiding cues and niches for immune cells. Due to its assembly together with other extracellular matrix molecules such as collagens, tenascin-C forms matrix tracks that presumably create sites of high local tissue stiffness which could have an impact on cellular signaling and may promote metastasis similarly as was shown for a stiffened collagen matrix (Leventhal et al., 2009). Tenascin-C matrix tracks can form channels and presumably form niches for disseminated cancer cells as had been seen in melanomas. Tenascin-C attracts endothelial cells to form sprouts, yet in tenascin-C matrix tracks no endothelial cells are found. These observations are in agreement with a potential dual impact of tenascin-C on angiogenesis; a tenascin-C matrix might stimulate sprouting, yet at a high local tenascin-C concentration anoikis in endothelial cells might be induced due to its anti-adhesive properties. In consequence vessels might undergo pruning leaving remnants of tenascin-C matrix that upon remodelling by adjacent tumor and tumor associated cells gives rise to the observed matrix tracks. Cells may receive signals from a tenascin-C substratum through receptor mediated interactions involving several integrins such as $\alpha v \beta 3$, $\alpha v \beta 6$ and $\alpha 9 \beta 1$. Integrin signaling also might be triggered indirectly, in particular in a fibronectin context (fibronectin is part of the tenascin-C matrix tracks, see Figure 3) through masking syndecan-4 binding sites in fibronectin thus inhibiting signaling by an $\alpha 5 \beta 1$ integrin/syndecan-4 complex. Tenascin-C binds growth factors which could activate or inhibit their signaling. Finally tenascin-C can enhance expression of genes such as MSI1 and LGR5 through yet unknown upstream events and thus may activate associated Wnt and Notch signaling, two pathways promoting angiogenesis and metastasis. Tenascin-C might alter the properties of the local tumor microenvironment/niche by blocking the expression of the LRP5/6 signaling inhibitor DKK1 thus creating a microenvironment that is permissive for LRP-dependent Wnt, TGFβ, PDGF, CTGF (and presumably other not yet identified LRP5/6 dependent) signaling that has been shown to promote angiogenesis and metastasis. It is intriguing to speculate that tenascin-C is part of a niche, a "soil", where pro-angiogenic and pro-metastatic signaling is promoted by releasing signaling inhibitor brakes (that have been presumably implemented as feedback loops to guarantee proper tissue homeostasis) by repression of these inhibitors..

In summary, tenascin-C seems to promote metastasis by different poorly understood mechanisms. Tenascin-C expression by either tumor or stromal cells in the primary tumor promotes cancer cell dissemination and survival in the circulation. A promoting role of tenascin-C on proliferation, migration, invasion and EMT and the formation of particular tenascin-C rich matrix channels is in agreement with this concept. Moreover, in addition to the expression of tenascin-C in the primary tumor early expression of tenascin-C by tumor cells and later expression by stromal cells also plays a crucial role in metastasis. Recent publications suggest a role for tenascin-C in cooperating with other extracellular matrix molecules in inducing pro-metastatic signaling (e.g. Notch and Wnt signaling) that would promote the survival and colonization of cancer cells at the metastatic site. A graphical summary is provided in Figure 4. Despite these important insights it is still an enigma how tenascin-C in the primary tumor can impact on the pre-metastatic niche. Which domains of tenascin-C and which tenascin-C receptors are involved? Which effects are triggered by a direct contact of tenascin-C with the cells, which effects are indirect and mediated by alterations in tissue organization and stiffness? How are the identified tenascin-C linked signaling pathways regulated by tenascin-C? For addressing these questions more appropriate 3D co-culture models with defined tenascin-C subdomain molecules and immune competent tumor models with a defined tenascin-C expression and a stochastic development of tumors and metastasis are needed.

# Chapter 4

# Clinical Impact

Cancer is a leading cause of death in humans with a high complexity and often patient-specific etiopathology. It therefore requires the development of new and advanced strategies for anti-cancer treatment. The most commonly used ways to treat cancer are resection, radiation and chemotherapy. Whereas in some cancer types these treatments are highly effective, other tumor types are resistant to cytotoxic agents or ionizing radiation and severe side-effects to intact organs frequently occur. In the meantime, new concepts have been developed such as vaccination, the use of antibodies, peptides, nucleic acids or protein inhibitors to target cancer-specific signaling pathways or proteins, including tenascin-C.

## 4.1  Targeting Tenascin-C in Cancer

Extensive research over the past 30 years since its discovery, the most recent of which has been summarized in the preceding sections in this book, has shown that tenascin-C plays an important role in different phases of tumorigenesis and tumor progression. In contrast to most adult tissues where tenascin-C is absent tenascin-C becomes highly expressed in almost all solid cancers (and some leukemias) where its high expression levels correlate with cancer progression and a poor prognosis in some cancers. High tenascin-C levels are found at the invasive front of carcinomas and correlate with abundance of tumor blood vessels and metastasis to lymph nodes and distant organs. Tenascin-C promotes survival, proliferation and migration and thus appears to contribute to most of the six proposed hallmarks of cancer (Hanahan and Weinberg, 2011). Although analysis of human cancer tissue rather implicated a role for tenascin-C in cancer progression there is evidence (mostly from murine tumor models) that also early events such as cell survival and proliferation within the primary tumor and the angiogenic switch are regulated and promoted by tenascin-C. Expression of the tenascin-C molecule is regulated by alternative splicing, glycosylation and proteolytic cleavage, thus generating a multitude of different molecules with quite distinct (not well understood) functions, yet these molecules are all covered by the name tenascin-C. Tenascin-C binds several extracellular matrix molecules and together these molecules form distinct fibrillar networks that not only generate physical and local niches representing particular microenvironments but presumably also impact on tissue stiffness, associated cellular signaling, angiogenesis and tumor cell dissemination. A substratum of purified tenascin-C is anti-adhesive for most cells in culture and tenascin-C can reduce the adhesive strength of fibronectin (and maybe other not yet identified extracellular matrix molecules). Tenascin-C binds cell surface receptors such as integrin $\alpha v\beta 3$, EGFR and TLR4 and triggers cellular signaling and in case of TLR4 secretion of pro-inflammatory cytokines. Tenascin-C also alters cellular signaling by non-receptor directed interactions through competitive binding to fibronectin thus blocking the integrin adhesion co-receptor function of syndecan-4, leading to impaired actin stress fiber formation and reduced cell spreading on fibronectin. Through its impact on the actin cytoskeleton tenascin-C can regulate cellular signaling leading to specific gene expression (as e.g. down regulation of DKK1). In addition, tenascin-C also binds soluble pro-angiogenic and pro-tumorigenic factors and thus may create a gradient of soluble factors. By sequestration and/or presentation tenascin-C may regulate signaling induced by these factors, yet it is currently unknown whether this would promote or inhibit the activity of these molecules (both is likely). It is conceivable that tenascin-C provides a signaling permissive microenvironment by repression of DKK1 which occurs in several cells within a tumor, thus presumably relieving several LRP5/6 dependent pro-angiogenic/pro-tumorigenic signaling pathways from inhibition by DKK1. Signaling pathways that are regulated by tenascin-C have already been identified and it appears that responses to tenascin-C are cell type and context dependent. Altogether our understanding about the role of tenascin-C is still limited due to its enigmatic form-to-function relation, its multiple and complex interactions with cells, and with other extracellular matrix and soluble molecules that we only begin to understand. Yet, its high expression in cancer tissue makes tenascin-C a very promising target for novel diagnostic and therapeutic approaches in anti-cancer therapy. This is evidenced by numerous filed patents which protect the use of specific tenascin-C domains, the production and use of monoclonal antibodies against specific domains of tenascin-C or the development of novel therapeutic concepts (based on nucleic acids) for targeting tenascin-C expression or the tenascin-C molecule itself as tumor specific address. In the following section, we will summarize some of the most advanced strategies that had been developed for anti-cancer treatment by targeting tenascin-C. Some of these strategies already have advanced into clinical testing (see Table 8).

## 4.2   Anti-tenascin-C Antibodies in Anti-cancer Therapy

The generation of monoclonal antibodies with strong affinities to a specific molecule is the most applied strategy in the development of novel anti-cancer drugs. Such antibodies can be modified and coupled with cytotoxic agents such as cytokines. Several antibodies, mostly recognizing isoforms of tenascin-C containing the alternatively spliced domains A1 to D, have been developed and a few have been examined in preclinical or clinical trials (Table 8, Figure 5). A detailed summary of the use of anti-tenascin-C antibodies in radiotherapy of cancer can be found in the book "Monoclonal Antibody and Peptide-Targeted Radiotherapy of Cancer" (Reilly, 2010).

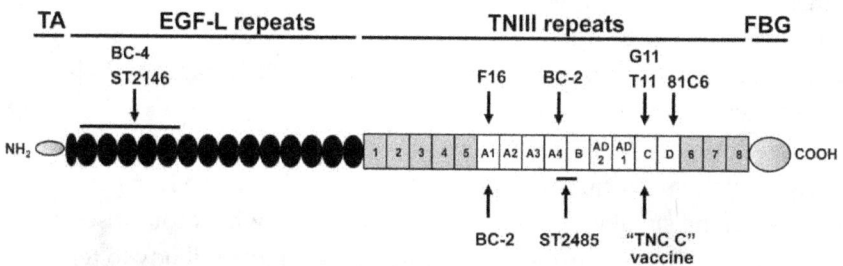

Figure 5: Overview of monoclonal antibodies and vaccine generated for targeting tenascin-C in anti-cancer treatment. Black arrows indicate the specific tenascin-C targeting domain of the different antibodies. "TNC C" vaccine is based on a fusion protein of thioredoxin and a peptide comprising TNIII C repeat. A detailed summary including references can be found in Table 8.

The monoclonal antibody **81C6** was generated from mice which were immunized with the glioma cell line U-251 MG. It exhibits specific binding to tenascin-C of different cancer types including glioma (Bourdon *et* *al.*, 1983) and specifically targets TNIII-domain C/D (Bourdon *et al.*, 1985). The potential of this antibody in cancer therapeutics for delivery of radioisotopes was tested in the 1980s in subcutaneous and intracranial xenograft mouse models of glioma. Intravenous injection of iodine labeled 81C6-[131]I inhibited tumor growth compared to non-specific isotype control antibody (Lee *et al.*, 1988a; Lee *et al.*, 1988b). After improvement of this antibody leading to higher tumor accumulation and enhanced stability (Sampson *et al.*, 2006) several phase I and II clinical trials were performed to determine dose, efficacy and toxicity on glioma patients with the purpose to target remaining tumor cells after resection. 81C6-[131]I was delivered by injection into the surgically created resection cavity followed by either fixed radiotherapy dosing (Reardon *et al.*, 2006) or patient-specific 44-Gy boost (Reardon *et al.*, 2008). Another phase I study used alpha-particle-emitting radionuclide [211]At with shorter range and more potent cytotoxicity. 81C6 coupled to [211]At (81C6-[211]At) was injected into the resection cavity of glioma patients (Zalutsky *et al.*, 2008). So far, these three studies showed safe administration of radionuclide coupled 81C6 with low toxicity and survival benefit in some patients but a significant therapeutic improvement could not be observed in the low numbers of patients included in the studies. A follow up phase III clinical trial for combination therapy of 81C6-[131]I with Temozolomide and radiotherapy after tumor resection was planned but terminated due to funding issues. Another phase II trial for combination therapy with the anti-angiogenic drug Bevacizumab was requested by Bradmer Pharmaceuticals but the status is currently unknown.

The company Philogen developed a fully humanized antibody called "**F16**" which specifically recognizes the TNIII-domain A1 of tenascin-C. Injected in the small immunoprotein (SIP) format, which comprises a protein fragment derived from the variable region of an antibody to tenascin-C, in a brain cancer xenograft model, the antibody accumulated selectively in the tumor but not in other organs (Brack *et al.*, 2006). Using this antibody for tissue staining showed tenascin-C expression in many different human cancer types such as in lymphoma (Schliemann *et al.*, 2009), renal cell carcinoma (Berndt *et al.*, 2010), lung cancer (Pedretti *et al.*, 2009), head and neck cancer (Schwager *et al.*, 2011), glioblastoma multiforme (GBM) (Pedretti *et al.*, 2010) and melanoma (Frey *et al.*, 2011) suggesting a potential application in many cancer types. The antibody was coupled to interleukin-2 (IL2) with the aim to improve classical treatment such as chemotherapy by using tenascin-C as tumor specific address for delivery of IL2 to attract the immune system to eliminate the tumor cells.

IL2 is approved for treatment of cancer (Proleukin®, Novartis) and shows activity against renal cell carcinoma, melanoma, lymphoma or leukemia. Applied in the conjugated scFv format (**F16-IL2**, Teleukin) in a breast cancer xenograft model in combination with the chemotherapeutic agents paclitaxel or doxorubicin showed a significant reduced tumor volume as compared to single treatment with IL2 or chemotherapy alone (Marlind *et al.*, 2008). The antibody was also tested in preclinical models of brain cancer together with standard chemotherapy of Temozolomide. The combined treatment led to complete tumor remission in animals with subcutaneous tumors. In an orthotopic setting of that combination therapy, tumors were 70 % smaller and the survival rate of the animals was prolonged from 3 to about 6 months (Pedretti *et al.*, 2010). These results reveal reasonable effects in murine tumor models and prospects of applicability in human cancer patients due to recognition of tenascin-C in human cancer tissue by the F16 antibody. Indeed, recently, application of F16-IL2 in combination with cytarabine was described in a single patient with acute myeloid leukemia (AML) (Gutbrodt *et al.*, 2013). This patient previously relapsed from multiple therapeutic approaches. The patient received F16-IL2 (30 MIU day 1, 50 MIU day 8, intravenously) and dytarabine (5 mg twice daily on days 1 to 10, subcutaneously). Additional local radiotherapy of some AML lesions was performed to improve difficulties in swallowing and vessel compression. The authors describe an immediate symptomatic improvement shortly after therapy was started and even before the first application of radiotherapy. PET/CT imaging at day 14 showed a nearly complete disappearance of AML lesions after 2 weeks of treatment (Gutbrodt *et al.*, 2013). Currently, a phase I/II clinical trial is in progress in patients with solid tumors (including breast and lung cancer) where F16-IL2 is applied together with paclitaxel or doxorubicine. First results from phase Ib trials showed that the combined treatment can safely be administered with disease stabilization in a few cases (De Braud *et al.*, 2011). Another clinical trial was recently initiated to evaluate a potential application of F16-IL2 together with paclitaxel in metastatic Merkel cell carcinoma (EudraCT: 2012-004018-33).

The F16 antibody is also tested for a possible use in targeted radionuclide therapy. F16-SIP was labeled with iodine [124]I (**[124]I-F16SIP**) injected into 4 patients with head and neck cancer following immuno-PET imaging. Beside an antibody uptake in several secondary organs a tumor-specific signal was visible in all patients 24 hours after injection (Heuveling *et al.*, 2013). Another phase I/II clinical trial is currently ongoing using F16 coupled to iodine [131]I ([131]I-F16SIP, Tenarad) for radiotherapy in several cancer types. Administration of [131]I-F16SIP to a low number of Hodgkin's lymphoma patients refractory to conventional treatment showed acceptable toxicity such as hematologic toxicity at grade 3 or lower. Some of the patients even showed disease stabilization with a reduced number and/or size of lesions (Aloj *et al.*, 2011). These examples demonstrate tolerance, bioavailability and possible selective tumor targeting of the radionuclide labeled F16 antibody which needs further clinical exploration on larger patient cohorts.

A few other monoclonal antibodies (G11, T11, ST2146, ST2185, BC-2, BC-4) have been raised against tenascin-C for a cancer-specific radionuclide delivery. Some of them were modified to reach higher purity levels for pharmaceutical use or techniques have been developed to enhance sensitivity of current applications. Some of these antibody-based methods are listed in Table 8, but are not discussed in more detail here. Currently, none of them reached clinical trials beyond phase II. For the moment, antibody-based cancer-therapeutics targeting tenascin-C have only been tested in phase I/II clinical trials for safety, dose and toxicity issues using small patient cohorts, mainly suffering from brain tumors. Most of these studies show that the agents can be safely administered and some indicate that the developed strategy might be beneficial in severe cases of cancer which are refractory to conventional therapies which can be envisioned to be beneficial in particular in combination with cytotoxic drugs. In summary, these results underpin the importance and feasibility of a targeting strategy using tenascin-C expression as address. Studies on larger patient cohorts need to be performed to evaluate a potential applicability of this antibody strategy in the clinic.

## 4.3 Nucleic Acid-based Strategies for Recognition of Tenascin-C in Cancer Tissue

The development of nucleic acid-based strategies is an alternative to the use of antibodies as cancer therapeutics. Such novel drugs include ribozymes, small interfering RNAs (siRNA) or aptamers which are already in clinical trials for different pathologies, including cancer (Burnett and Rossi, 2012). Here, the development of nucleic acid based drugs for tenascin-C will be described.

| Compound | Strategy | Cancer type | Latest clinical stage | Observation | Reference |
|---|---|---|---|---|---|
| | | Antibody-based | | | |
| 81C6-[131]I (Neuradiab) | Regional targeted radiotherapy; Injection into cavity after resection; | Glioma | Phase I/II | Feasible, No/low toxicity, Non-significant but encouraging overall outcome | (Reardon et al., 2006; Reardon et al., 2008) |
| 81C6-[211]At | Co-treatment with chemotherapy | | | | (Zalutsky et al., 2008) |
| 81C6-[131]I (Neuradiab) | Co-treatment with Bevacizumab | Glioma | Phase II | Unknown trial status | NCT00906516 |
| F16-IL2 (Teleukin) | Co-treatment with Temozolomide | U87 (GBM) | Preclinical | Growth inhibition; Survival prolongation | (Pedretti et al., 2010) |
| | Co-treatment with Cytarabine | Acute myeloid leukemia | Treatment of one patient | Rapid disappearance of AML lesions, improved clinical symptoms | (Gutbrodt et al., 2013) |
| | Co-treatment with Doxorubicine | MDA-MB231; Advanced solid tumors; | Phase Ib/II (2008-2013) NCT01131364 | Safe administration; disease stabilization | (De Braud et al., 2011; Marlind et al., 2008) |
| | Co-treatment with Paclitaxel | Breast cancer, Lung cancer | Phase Ib/II (2008-2013) NCT01134250 | | |
| | Co-treatment with Paclitaxel | Melanoma (metastatic Merkel cell carcinoma) | Phase II (started 2013) | - | 2012-004018-33 (EudraCT) |

| | | | | | |
|---|---|---|---|---|---|
| F16-$^{131}$I (Tenarad) | Radionuclide therapy | Hodgkin's disease, Solid tumors | Phase Ib/II NCT01240720 | Good partial response, stabilization of Hodgkin's disease | (Aloj et al., 2011) |
| F16-$^{124}$I | Radionuclide therapy | Head and neck cancer | Phase 0 | Good tolerance, bio-available, tumor-specific uptake | (Heuveling et al., 2013) |
| BC-2-$^{131}$I, BC-4-$^{131}$I | Regional targeted radiotherapy | Glioma | Phase II | Stabilization, partial or complete remission | (Riva et al., 1994) |
| BC-4-biotin + avidin + $^{99}$Y-biotin | Pre-targeted Antibody-Guided RadioImmuno-Therapy (PAGRIT) | Glioma | Phase I | Stabilization or partial remission | (Paganelli et al., 2001) |
| ST2146, ST2185 | PAGRIT; combination of anti-tenascin-C antibodies | HT-29 (colon), U-118 (brain) | Preclinical | Tumor-specific localization | (De Santis et al., 2006; Petronzelli et al., 2005) |
| G11, G11-IL2 | mAb generation targeting TNIII C- domain | Lung, brain | Preclinical | Tumor-specific localization | (Silacci et al., 2006) |
| TN11 | mAb generation targeting TNIII C-domain | - | - | Suitable for histological staining (breast, brain cancer) | (Carnemolla et al., 1999) |
| Nucleic-acid based | | | | | |
| anti-TNC dsRNA (ATN-RNA) | Interference RNA intervention | Brain cancer | 46 patients after tumor resection | Prolonged survival; Improved quality of life | (Rolle et al., 2010) |

| | Therapeutic strategy | Cancer type | Clinical stage | Main observations | Reference |
|---|---|---|---|---|---|
| Aptamer $^{99m}$Tc-TTA1 | Targeted radiotherapy | Various xenograft models | Preclinical | Tumor-specific uptake | (Hicke et al., 2001; Hicke et al., 2006; Schmidt et al., 2004) |
| Aptamer GBI-10 | Aptamer generation by SELEX to target tenascin-C | - | - | Interaction with several tenascin-C peptides | (Daniels et al., 2003) |
| SMART Simultaneous Multiple Aptamers and RGD Targeting | Nanoparticles coated with aptamers and peptides targeting nucleolin, tenascin-C and RGD at once | Several human cancer cell lines | - | Enhanced sensitivity compared to mono-targeting strategy | (Ko et al., 2011) |
| Vaccination | | | | | |
| TRX-TNC C | Fusion proteins of thioredoxin with tumor vessel specific antigens (TNC C domain, FN-EDA, FN-EDB, ANXA1, CD248, MR) | Subcutaneous mouse xenograft; spontaneous Rip1-Tag2 model | Preclinical | High anti-TNC antibody titers in immunized mice or rabbits; Reduced tumor volume (FN-EDB) | (Huijbers, 2012; Huijbers et al., 2010; Olsson and Hellman, 2011) |

**Table 8:** Overview of strategies for tenascin-C targeted cancer therapeutics. For each approach, the compound name, its envisaged therapeutic strategy and targeting cancer type is listed. The last known clinical stage and short summary of main observations which can be found in the indicated references are specified. NCT and EudraCT identifiers are indicated for clinical studies listed on webpage "ClinicalTrials.gov" and "eudract.ema.europa.eu".

**Aptamers** are short oligonucleotides with specific binding to a target molecule with very high affinity and selectivity, similar to monoclonal antibodies (Tuerk *et al.*, 1992). The advantage of aptamers are several fold; they are stable and can be designed with desired length and specific binding affinities for a target molecule. Moreover, aptamers can be linked to other molecules such as cytokines and thus can deliver molecules to specific molecular addresses within a given tissue similar to antibodies. Using the SELEX technology applied to U251 glioblastoma cells or purified tenascin-C protein, the aptamer "TTA1" was generated with a high specificity and selectivity for human tenascin-C (Hicke *et al.*, 2001). Further modifications improved biodistribution and led to the design of radionuclide-labeled [99]mTc-TTA1 that upon intravenous injection into nude mice showed a tumor specific accumulation in the human tumor cell xenograft of glioma (Schmidt *et al.*, 2004), colon, breast and rhabdomyosarcoma cells (Hicke *et al.*, 2006). Thus [99]mTc-TTA1 appears to be useful for targeting several human cancers. In the same group another aptamer was generated (**GBI-10**). Although *in vivo* studies are not published the authors present data where GBI-10 was used for affinity purification of target proteins. Liquid chromatography tandem mass spectroscopy revealed the interaction of GBI-10 with several tenascin-C peptides. These were located along the whole protein demonstrating target-specific binding of the aptamer to several sites within tenascin-C (Daniels *et al.*, 2003).

Recently, Ko and colleagues further extended the aptamer approach and generated a multimodal nanoparticle-based <u>S</u>imultaneously <u>M</u>ultiple <u>A</u>ptamers and <u>R</u>GD <u>T</u>argeting (**SMART**) probe targeting nucleolin, integrin αvβ3 and tenascin-C at once. Compared to single-target probes TTA1, RGD or AS1411 the multi-target probe SMART provided a strongly enhanced specificity and binding intensity when applied to different human cancer cells *in vitro*. These included C6 glioma, DU145 prostate, HeLa cervical, NPA thyroid papillary and A549 non-small lung cancer cell lines (Ko *et al.*, 2011). However, no proof-of-concept has yet been performed in a pre-clinical *in vivo* model.

Compared to using radionuclide-labeled monoclonal antibodies, aptamers might be advantageous as they are smaller, can be produced by chemical synthesis in higher yields and product reproducibility and thus may be cheaper than antibodies. As has been shown for example with GBI-10, aptamers can also have several binding sites within the target protein whereas monoclonal antibodies only bind to one specific sequence. This could be particularly relevant in the case of tenascin-C with its multiple splice variants. Other advantages of aptamers are that they can be modified to improve their pharmacological properties, their resistance to degradation or to delay their renal elimination (Burnett and Rossi, 2012).

## 4.4   Nucleic Acid-based Strategies to Reduce Tenascin-C Expression in Cancer

Interesting results for a potential use of **RNA interference** (RNAi) to reduce tenascin-C in cancer tissue was demonstrated for the first time by Barciszewski and colleagues in human glioma patients (Rolle *et al.*, 2010; Wyszko *et al.*, 2008; Zukiel *et al.*, 2006). In the latest study 46 patients (grade II, III and IV) were injected with **ATN-RNA**, a double stranded RNA homologous to tenascin-C mRNA, into areas of neoplastic infiltration after resection of the primary tumor or upon resection of a recurrent tumor (Rolle *et al.*, 2010). Tumor growth was followed by MRI or CT imaging and survival rates were compared to 48 patients which had obtained brachytherapy (radiation). This comparison showed that ATN-RNA application prolonged survival by a median of 4.8 weeks (grade II from 176.1 to 180.9 weeks), 13.2 weeks (grade III from 59.1 to 72.3 weeks) and 13.9 weeks in glioma patients with grade IV disease (from 52.8 to 66.7 weeks). The ATN-RNA administration further had improved quality of life as determined by the Karnofsky Performance Scale. A beneficial effect was even more obvious for patients with recurrent tumors (Rolle *et al.*, 2010). Although the authors claim that the use of dsRNA ATN-RNA has many advantages in terms of natural target for RISC, as e.g. absence of interferon induction, no requirement of further stabilization and no off-target effects (Rolle *et al.*, 2010), knock down of tenascin-C will only occur transiently at the site of injection and therefore needs repetitive administration with unknown side effects and high costs. Beside these first promising results it is conceivable that the development of a long-lasting knock down of tenascin-C with systematic administration could be successful in reducing tenascin-C expression in glioblastoma. But for this several issues need to be solved as mentioned above including sufficient delivery to sites of high tenascin-C expression.

## 4.5   Vaccination

The development of therapeutic vaccines for treating existing tumors is another novel approach in cancer-treatment and many vaccines are currently tested in clinical trials for different cancer types. To date, only two therapeutic vaccines are approved. One by the FDA for use in patients with metastatic prostate cancer (Gardner *et al.*, 2012) and another one exclusively in Russia for the treatment of patients with recurrent kidney cancer (Wood *et al.*, 2008). These are still cost-intensive procedures which require patient-specific isolation and *ex-vivo* processing of cells or proteins to generate the custom-made vaccine.

A novel and custom made vaccination approach targeting several tumor specific antigens, including TNIII C-domain, is currently under development by Olsson and colleagues which was recently protected by a patent (Olsson and Hellman, 2011). This strategy is based on six different antigens which are preferentially expressed in the tumor vasculature but not in healthy tissue or normal blood vessels: fibronectin extra-domains A and B (FN-EDA, FN-EDB), extra-domain C of tenascin-C (**TNC C**), annexin A1, endosialin (CD248) and magic roundabout (MR). The invention contains the development of a vaccine using one or a combination of these proteins which are modified in a way that the immune system recognizes the modified self-protein as a non-self protein. To date, the *in vivo* proof of concept was only shown for FN-EDB. A fusion protein between the 91 amino acid long FN-EDB and *E.coli* thioredoxin was generated (TRX-EDB) and injected into mice which then showed high titers of anti-EDB antibodies. Then, T241 fibrosarcoma cells were grafted subcutaneously into these mice. Mice treated with TRX-EDB developed much smaller and highly necrotic tumors which lacked a structured organization compared to a control group. Consistently, tumor vessels showed an altered morphology and the presence of macrophages within the endothelium indicated destruction of the blood vessels by the immune system (Huijbers *et al.*, 2010). Furthermore, vaccination of mice and rabbits against **TNC C** showed the presence of TNC C-specific antibodies in serum of these animals. A combination therapy against EDA, EDB and TNC C together is currently under investigation and will be tested in xenograft experiments or models of spontaneous tumor formation.

The strategy was further applied in a second independent model of spontaneous tumor formation. Upon immunization against FN-EDB, PNET/Rip1Tag2 mice showed a reduced number of pancreatic tumors compared to control animals (Huijbers, 2012). This tumor model better mimics tumor formation in humans than xenografts in immune compromised mice. Compared to the use of monoclonal antibodies, the vaccination approach would overcome cost-intensive repetitive injections as the organism produces an immune response and the tumor antigen specific antibodies by itself. This approach may even allow vaccination against several tumor antigens simultaneously.

## 4.6 Tenascin-C and its Value in Cancer Prediction, Treatment and Diagnosis

As described in detail in Chapter 1 tenascin-C is highly expressed in most malignant solid tumors and some leukemias (Orend and Chiquet-Ehrismann, 2006) as evidenced by strong tissue staining and high mRNA expression levels in cancer tissue. As a potential prognostic marker its presence was also analyzed in body liquids and it could be detected in serum of patients with several cancers such as colorectal carcinoma (Riedl *et al.*, 1995; Takeda *et al.*, 2007), malignant melanoma (Burchardt *et al.*, 2003), pancreatic cancer (Esposito *et al.*, 2006) or non-small cell lung cancer (Ishiwata *et al.*, 2005). Unfortunately, tenascin-C in serum is a questionable general tumor marker as many patients display normal tenascin-C levels which do not correlate with tumor progression. Moreover, in prostate cancer tenascin-C serum levels rather correlate with signs of inflammation and infection than with cancer (Schenk *et al.*, 1995).

However, tenascin-C still may become a valid predictive marker in some cancer types as its high expression in the tumor tissue often correlates with poor prognosis or metastasis (Orend and Chiquet-Ehrismann, 2006) (Table 1, Table 6). Here we discuss GBM as the cancer type for which specific tenascin-C expression has been most exploited as unique tool for imaging or treatment.

GBM is one of the most aggressive tumors with poor prognosis. In glioma patients, high stromal tenascin-C expression levels were associated with tumor invasion and shorter disease-free survival (Leins *et al.*, 2003). Surgery and radiotherapy have only a short benefit on overall survival of GBM patients and tumors often re-grow after resection. Due to strong vascularization of these tumors anti-angiogenic therapies are currently under clinical testing (Chi *et al.*, 2009). Phase I/II clinical trials using Bevacizumab (Avastin®, Genentech), a monoclonal antibody targeting VEGFA, demonstrated biological activity in recurrent GBM (Friedman *et al.*, 2009; Kreisl *et al.*, 2009). A combination therapy of Bevacizumab with Irinotecan, compared to Bevacizumab alone, improved 6-month progression-free survival rates from 42.6% to 50.3% and the median overall survival from 8.7 to 9.2 months (Friedman *et al.*, 2009). Yet, a significant number of patients did not respond to the treatment (Vredenburgh *et al.*, 2007) or even showed tumor regrowth and accelerated clinical decline after drug withdrawal (Zuniga *et al.*, 2010). It seems that the use of anti-angiogenic treatment is questionable in some cancer patients with GBM and may even worsen prognosis.

This was further investigated in different *in vivo* tumor models. Anti-angiogenic tumor therapies targeting VEGF receptor signaling showed beneficial anti-tumor effects but at the same time it accelerated metastasis formation and decreased survival (Ebos *et al.*, 2009) or it increased tumor invasiveness and supported the formation of local and distant metastasis (Paez-Ribes *et al.*, 2009) after drug withdrawal. It was observed that after anti-angiogenic treatment endothelial cells were eliminated but that empty sleeves of extracellular matrix comprising collagen IV remained intact. It was further shown that these matrix sleeves provided a scaffold for rapid revascularization upon end of treatment (Mancuso *et al.*, 2006). Lumen forming tube-like structures rich of extracellular matrix have already been described elsewhere and it is speculated that they could serve as scaffold for tumor cell dissemination. Tube-like extracellular matrix structures contain tenascin-C in melanoma (Kaariainen *et al.*, 2006; Maniotis *et al.*, 1999) and in Rip1Tag2 tumors (our unpublished data) and were seen in conduits of the thymus and lymph nodes (Drumea-Mirancea *et al.*, 2006). We had previously speculated that a genetic program for the formation of tenascin-C-rich conduits in secondary lymphoid organs potentially is turned on in cancer (Midwood and Orend, 2009). Thus, tenascin-C could be a therapeutic target to counteract the rebound effect, revascularization and tumor progression in GBM after discontinuation of the anti-angiogenic treatment or resistance development.

The different strategies presented above might also become useful for non-invasive *in situ* tumor detection by MRI, PET or ultrasound imaging, techniques by which tumors only bigger than 1 cm can be detected (Weissleder, 2006). Molecular imaging is becoming increasingly important in cancer diagnosis by using cancer-specific target-based imaging probes. Using probes coupled to fluorescent dyes or radioisotopes *in vivo* had been shown in preclinical models (Banerjee *et al.*, 2010; Shah *et al.*, 2009). The monoclonal antibodies 81C6 and F16 (Frey *et al.*, 2011; Schwager *et al.*, 2011), aptamer TTA1 (Hicke *et al.*, 2006) and the multi-target strategy SMART (Ko *et al.*, 2011) may provide perspectives for live imaging of tumors for an improved early detection of metastasis.

Most of the above mentioned monoclonal antibodies are specific for the large tenascin-C isoform. However, monospecificity to a single domain, antibody size or not fully humanized molecules might be disadvantageous for some cancer types. Here, other approaches such as the use of aptamers, RNAi or vaccination might be more useful since the production is easier and cheaper and multi-targeting approaches are possible. Unfortunately, advanced clinical trials are still missing. More-over, an increased knowledge about the tumor-, patient- and stage-specific expression of tenascin-C and its splice variants is required to develop more specific and flexible therapies for targeting tenascin-C. These approaches may be useful to be applied upon development of resistance against cytotoxic or anti-angiogenic drugs.

# Chapter 5

# Conclusions and Future Perspectives

Since the discovery of tenascin-C 30 years ago, and the subsequent early studies in murine models which provided the first indication that targeting tenascin-C in tumors may have significant therapeutic benefit, what we know about how this molecule acts within the tumor extracellular matrix, and at the metastatic site, has advanced considerably. This is reflected in the sheer volume of peer reviewed journal articles and patents that detail the promise of this approach. However, what is also clear is that none of these approaches (except one anecdotal case in an AML patient) have yet yielded a proven mode of treatment effective in tumor types characterized by elevated tenascin-C expression. The recent data that we have highlighted in this book exemplifies the vast complexity of tenascin-C expression, splicing and cell type specific effects of this extracellular matrix molecule. A greater understanding of precisely how tenascin-C works within a complex, 3D extracellular matrix to control tumor behavior is needed. The contribution of tenascin-C to metastasis must also be deciphered in more detail, since it becomes apparent that targeting the primary tumor alone is not optimally effective. Moreover, the tumor specific nature of the role of tenascin-C must be elucidated to enable the tailoring of appropriate treatments to the correct patient subsets.

Tenascin-C is highly conserved throughout evolution of mammals and rarely has been seen to have mutations. This argues for a selective pressure that maintains this molecule in its once evolved form. But why is that? Does tenascin-C play predominantly a structural/architectural role or does it modulate and counter balance other extracellular matrix molecules? If so these functions are apparently important. Maybe tenascin-C has even adopted another life-saving function due to its "stickiness" as exemplified by sequestering HIV and thus enabling its elimination (Fouda *et al.*, 2013). Maybe this applies to other viruses and pathogens? In this context it would be interesting to exploit the HIV sequestration function of tenascin-C for anti-cancer treatment or diagnosis as was speculated above.

The enigma of the form-to-function relationship of tenascin-C is one of the most important obstacles to understand the roles of tenascin-C in cancer and other diseases. It is also the most difficult to address in particular given that within tissues several cell types may express tenascin-C with different domain compositions. If we knew how tenascin-C expression is regulated at transcriptional and splicing level we could design strategies to normalize tenascin-C expression in cancer tissue (Tucker and Chiquet-Ehrismann, 2009). We are also ignorant about how glycosylation affects the conformation and function of tenascin-C which could have an impact on binding of tenascin-C to other extracellular matrix molecules and HIV (and maybe other pathogens). Tenascin-C is expressed in normal tissues at a few places (e.g. in stem cell niches, thymus, spleen, underneath the basement membrane of some epithelia) and, in cancer as tumor matrix tracks (Tucker and Chiquet-Ehrismann, 2009). What is tenascin-C doing there? Does tenascin-C affect extracellular matrix network formation in stem cell niches and in cancer? Due to its multivalent character (multiple domains, hexabrachion) it is possible that tenascin-C serves as a platform to organize extracellular matrix networks. On the contrary tenascin-C might also disturb normal matrix organization thus leading to altered networks as e.g. found in the tenascin-C matrix tracks of cancer tissue. Can we learn something about its role in network formation by analysing tenascin-C networks in the conduits of the thymus and the reticular fibers of the spleen? Given its high abundance in cancer tissue it is likely that the tenascin-C matrix tracks will have an impact on tissue stiffness and through that on the biomechanical properties of cancer tissue and cellular signaling. But this has not been addressed so far and is also not an easy task. Novel 3D cell culture models (as e.g. cell derived matrices, spheroids) and imaging techniques such as CLEM (correlative light and electron microscopy) and live imaging need to be adapted/applied to tackle the form-to-function enigma of tenascin-C.

Tenascin-C binds several soluble factors and by that tenascin-C rich extracellular matrices may create gradients of these factors within the cancer tissue. We had just started to see that a couple of soluble factors bind to tenascin-C (De Laporte *et al.*, 2013; Saupe *et al.*, 2013), but how many more factors would there be? How would the interaction be regulated? Does binding of soluble factors to tenascin-C enhance or inhibit the signaling activity of these factors? Tenascin-C is also processed by proteases. Does this have an impact on binding of soluble factors? Moreover, we just have started to get an idea that proteases can release anti- and pro-adhesive tenascin-C fragments (Ambort et al., 2010; Ruggiero et al., 2013). Would that apply to cancer? It would be important to understand how proteolytic cleavage of tenascin-C is regulated and what impact the fragments have on cellular signaling. Would they compete with full length tenascin-C or release cryptic interaction sites with novel functions?

In tumor tissue cells can interact with tenascin-C through cell surface receptors. At the same time cells may also receive information from soluble factors and other extracellular matrix molecules and we just have begun to understand that signals from soluble factors can have a huge impact on the adhesive properties of tenascin-C (Lange et al., 2007; Lange et al., 2008). It remains to be seen how these signals are integrated at cell level. Tenascin-C impacts on the actin cytoskeleton and it was just revealed that lack of actin stress fibers induced by tenascin-C inhibits gene expression of DKK1 (Saupe et al., 2013). What are the intracellular mediators? Tenascin-C also regulates miR expression (Piccinini and Midwood, 2012). Does modulation of the actin cytoskeleton by tenascin-C also regulates miR expression? And if so does this play a role in cancer?

The local microenvironment is believed to play an important role in cancer stemness that drives metastasis. Yet it remains an open question of how much of the stemness characteristic is encoded within the microenvironment and what is cell autonomous. Tenascin-C is expressed in angiogenic, metastatic and stem cell niches (Midwood et al., 2011). How tenascin-C contributes or even determines these niches and stemness properties of metastatic cancer cells is largely unknown.

Tenascin-C plays a role in adaptive and innate immunity and some underlying mechanisms just have been revealed. Knowing that the immune system is essential in cancer it remains to be seen how much knowledge acquired in immune compromised murine tumor models is relevant for understanding the role of tenascin-C in the human disease. An additional complication might arise from grafting human tumor cells into a murine host which may result in incompatibilities between the species specific microenvironments and thus may provide little useful information (Fantozzi and Christofori, 2006). In grafting models tumors develop much faster than in genetic tumor models and this has an impact on the formation of tumor specific extracellular matrix networks such as tenascin-C matrix tracks that are much less pronounced in grafted tumors. For all these reasons murine models with stochastic tumorigenesis and metastasis formation are needed where the tumor specific extracellular matrix (including high expression of tenascin-C) is phenocopied. The first murine tenascin-C transgenic tumor model just has recently been published and indeed had provided novel insights into the roles of tenascin-C in cancer. It was shown that tenascin-C is not only important in tumor progression (as expected from data in human cancer patients) but that tenascin-C also promotes early events of tumorigenesis such as enhancing tumor cell survival and proliferation as well as driving the angiogenic switch (Saupe *et al.*, 2013). This important information has been elapsed in the former studies but may be important for using tenascin-C expression in anti-cancer diagnosis and therapy.

Often, knockout mice are used to address the role of a molecule that is over expressed in pathological situations. The question arises whether this is a useful and appropriate approach. In case of tenascin-C it is believed that the real function of tenascin-C can be revealed when the phenotype in the absence of tenascin-C is the opposite to the phenotype upon high expression of tenascin-C. But this view should be cautioned. As an example, high tenascin-C expression was shown to correlate with breast cancer lung metastasis suggestive of a metastasis promoting function of tenascin-C. Therefore, it was anticipated that in the absence of tenascin-C less lung metastases would arise. Indeed this was the case when breast cancer cells with lowered tenascin-C levels (tenascin-C knock down) had been grafted (O'Connell *et al.*, 2011; Tavazoie *et al.*, 2008). However in a MMTV/PyMT tumor context with stochastic tumorigenesis no obvious difference in tumor growth nor lung metastasis was seen and this result was believed at that time to show that tenascin-C is not important in cancer (Talts *et al.*, 1999). Similarly, the first TNCKO mouse published was viable and did not show an obvious aberrant developmental phenotype (Saga *et al.*, 1992). These results has prompted the generation of a second TNCKO mouse, yet again the expected dramatic abnormal developmental phenotype was not seen (Forsberg *et al.*, 1996). This was thought to demonstrate that tenascin-C is dispensable for life and pathologies such as cancer. Subsequently, public funding for research on tenascin-C was difficult to obtain for many years. Meanwhile several studies have revealed multiple deficits in TNCKO tissue recovery inflicted by various insults (Mackie and Tucker, 1999). Another example for confusing results from the TNCKO mouse was obtained when addressing the role of tenascin-C in atherosclerosis. Tenascin-C is highly expressed in atherosclerotic plaques suggesting a role of tenascin-C in promoting atherosclerosis. Yet in the TNCKO mouse an unexpected phenotype was observed. Upon a fatty diet in an APOE-KO context there were even more atherosclerotic plaques observed than in a tenascin-C wild type background and this result was interpreted to reveal a protective role of tenascin-C in athero-sclerosis (Wang *et al.*, 2012).

Meanwhile there is plenty of evidence that supports an important role of tenascin-C in development and diseases. We hypothesize that tenascin-C is indispensible for life (supported by its high conservation throughout evolution) and therefore intricate, yet not at all understood compensatory mechanisms are at work in the TNCKO mouse (reviewed in (Mackie and Tucker, 1999; Midwood *et al.*, 2011; Midwood and Orend, 2009). This may have consequences for the application of TNCKO mice. To fully understand the role of tenascin-C in diseases with an overexpres-sion of tenascin-C it is advisable to use mouse models which mimic high tenascin-C expression in addition to TNCKO models. Hopefully, within less than 30 years we are able to report on the answers to many of these questions and strategies targeting cancer based on high tenascin-C ex-pression may have entered the clinics.

# References

Abaskharoun, M., Bellemare, M., Lau, E., and Margolis, R. U. (2010). Glypican-1, phosphacan/receptor protein-tyrosine phosphatase-zeta/beta and its ligand, tenascin-C, are expressed by neural stem cells and neural cells derived from embryonic stem cells. ASN Neuro 2, e00039.

Adams, M., Jones, J. L., Walker, R. A., Pringle, J. H., and Bell, S. C. (2002). Changes in tenascin-C isoform expression in invasive and preinvasive breast disease. Cancer Res 62, 3289-3297.

Aloj, L., D'Ambrosio, L., Aurilio, M., Marreno, R., Neri, D., Menssen, H. D., Giovannoni, L., Di Gennaro, F., Caraco, C., Arcamone, M., et al. (2011). Preliminary evaluation of radioimmunotherapy with Tenarad, a I-131 labeled antibody fragment targeting the extra-domain A1 of tenascin-C, in patients with refractory Hodgkin lymphoma. J Clin Oncol 29: ASCO Annual Meeting 2011 Abstract 8063.

Alves, T. R., da Fonseca, A. C., Nunes, S. S., da Silva, A. O., Dubois, L. G., Faria, J., Kahn, S. A., Viana, N. B., Marcondes, J., Legrand, C., et al. (2011). Tenascin-C in the extracellular matrix promotes the selection of highly proliferative and tubulogenesis-defective endothelial cells. Exp Cell Res 317, 2073-2085.

Ambort, D., Brellier, F., Becker-Pauly, C., Stocker, W., Andrejevic-Blant, S., Chiquet, M., and Sterchi, E. E. (2010). Specific processing of tenascin-C by the metalloprotease meprinbeta neutralizes its inhibition of cell spreading. Matrix Biol 29, 31-42.

Amonkar, S. D., Bertenshaw, G. P., Chen, T. H., Bergstrom, K. J., Zhao, J., Seshaiah, P., Yip, P., and Mansfield, B. C. (2009). Development and preliminary evaluation of a multivariate index assay for ovarian cancer. PLoS One 4, e4599.

Asano, T., Iwasaki, N., Kon, S., Kanayama, M., Morimoto, J., Minami, A., and Uede, T. (2013). alpha9beta1 integrin acts as a critical intrinsic regulator of human rheumatoid arthritis. Rheumatology (Oxford).

Atula, T., Hedstrom, J., Finne, P., Leivo, I., Markkanen-Leppanen, M., and Haglund, C. (2003). Tenascin-C expression and its prognostic significance in oral and pharyngeal squamous cell carcinoma. Anticancer Res 23, 3051-3056.

Aukhil, I., Slemp, C. C., Lightner, V. A., Nishimura, K., Briscoe, G., and Erickson, H. P. (1990). Purification of hexabrachion (tenascin) from cell culture conditioned medium, and separation from a cell adhesion factor. Matrix 10, 98-111.

Balkwill, F. R., and Mantovani, A. (2012). Cancer-related inflammation: common themes and therapeutic opportunities. Semin Cancer Biol 22, 33-40.

Ballard, V. L., Sharma, A., Duignan, I., Holm, J. M., Chin, A., Choi, R., Hajjar, K. A., Wong, S. C., and Edelberg, J. M. (2006). Vascular tenascin-C regulates cardiac endothelial phenotype and neovascularization. Faseb J 20, 717-719.

Banerjee, S. R., Pullambhatla, M., Byun, Y., Nimmagadda, S., Green, G., Fox, J. J., Horti, A., Mease, R. C., and Pomper, M. G. (2010). 68Ga-labeled inhibitors of prostate-specific membrane antigen (PSMA) for imaging prostate cancer. J Med Chem 53, 5333-5341.

Barbolina, M. V., Liu, Y., Gurler, H., Kim, M., Kajdacsy-Balla, A. A., Rooper, L., Shepard, J., Weiss, M., Shea, L. D., Penzes, P., et al. (2012). Matrix rigidity activates Wnt signaling through down-regulation of Dickkopf-1 protein. J Biol Chem 288, 141-151.

Barker, N., van Es, J. H., Kuipers, J., Kujala, P., van den Born, M., Cozijnsen, M., Haegebarth, A., Korving, J., Begthel, H., Peters, P. J., and Clevers, H. (2007). Identification of stem cells in small intestine and colon by marker gene Lgr5. Nature 449, 1003-1007.

Behrem, S., Zarkovic, K., Eskinja, N., and Jonjic, N. (2005). Distribution pattern of tenascin-C in glioblastoma: correlation with angiogenesis and tumor cell proliferation. Pathol Oncol Res 11, 229-235.

Beiter, K., Hiendlmeyer, E., Brabletz, T., Hlubek, F., Haynl, A., Knoll, C., Kirchner, T., and Jung, A. (2005). beta-Catenin regulates the expression of tenascin-C in human colorectal tumors. Oncogene *24*, 8200-8204.

Bergers, G., and Benjamin, L. E. (2003). Tumorigenesis and the angiogenic switch. Nat Rev Cancer *3*, 401-410.

Berndt, A., Anger, K., Richter, P., Borsi, L., Brack, S., Silacci, M., Franz, M., Wunderlich, H., Gajda, M., Zardi, L., *et al.* (2006). Differential expression of tenascin-C splicing domains in urothelial carcinomas of the urinary bladder. J Cancer Res Clin Oncol *132*, 537-546.

Berndt, A., Kollner, R., Richter, P., Franz, M., Voigt, A., Berndt, A., Borsi, L., Giavazzi, R., Neri, D., and Kosmehl, H. (2010). A comparative analysis of oncofetal fibronectin and tenascin-C incorporation in tumour vessels using human recombinant SIP format antibodies. Histochem Cell Biol *133*, 467-475.

Bloom, L., Ingham, K. C., and Hynes, R. O. (1999). Fibronectin regulates assembly of actin filaments and focal contacts in cultured cells via the heparin-binding site in repeat III13. Mol Biol Cell *10*, 1521-1536.

Borgia, B., Roesli, C., Fugmann, T., Schliemann, C., Cesca, M., Neri, D., and Giavazzi, R. (2009). A proteomic approach for the identification of vascular markers of liver metastasis. Cancer Res *70*, 309-318.

Borsi, L., Carnemolla, B., Nicolo, G., Spina, B., Tanara, G., and Zardi, L. (1992). Expression of different tenascin isoforms in normal, hyperplastic and neoplastic human breast tissues. Int J Cancer *52*, 688-692.

Bos, P. D., Zhang, X. H., Nadal, C., Shu, W., Gomis, R. R., Nguyen, D. X., Minn, A. J., van de Vijver, M. J., Gerald, W. L., Foekens, J. A., and Massague, J. (2009). Genes that mediate breast cancer metastasis to the brain. Nature *459*, 1005-1009.

Bourdon, M. A., Matthews, T. J., Pizzo, S. V., and Bigner, D. D. (1985). Immunochemical and biochemical characterization of a glioma-associated extracellular matrix glycoprotein. J Cell Biochem *28*, 183-195.

Bourdon, M. A., and Ruoslahti, E. (1989). Tenascin mediates cell attachment through an RGD-dependent receptor. J Cell Biol *108*, 1149-1155.

Bourdon, M. A., Wikstrand, C. J., Furthmayr, H., Matthews, T. J., and Bigner, D. D. (1983). Human glioma-mesenchymal extracellular matrix antigen defined by monoclonal antibody. Cancer Res 43, 2796-2805.

Brack, S. S., Silacci, M., Birchler, M., and Neri, D. (2006). Tumor-targeting properties of novel antibodies specific to the large isoform of tenascin-C. Clin Cancer Res 12, 3200-3208.

Brellier, F., Hostettler, K., Hotz, H. R., Ozcakir, C., Cologlu, S. A., Togbe, D., Ryffel, B., Roth, M., and Chiquet-Ehrismann, R. (2011a). Tenascin-C triggers fibrin accumulation by downregulation of tissue plasminogen activator. FEBS Lett 585, 913-920.

Brellier, F., Ruggiero, S., Zwolanek, D., Martina, E., Hess, D., Brown-Luedi, M., Hartmann, U., Koch, M., Merlo, A., Lino, M., and Chiquet-Ehrismann, R. (2011b). SMOC1 is a tenascin-C interacting protein over-expressed in brain tumors. Matrix Biol 30, 225-233.

Brinckmann, J., Hunzelmann, N., Kahle, B., Rohwedel, J., Kramer, J., Gibson, M. A., Hubmacher, D., and Reinhardt, D. P. (2010). Enhanced fibrillin-2 expression is a general feature of wound healing and sclerosis: potential alteration of cell attachment and storage of TGF-beta. Lab Invest 90, 739-752.

Brunner, A., Mayerl, C., Tzankov, A., Verdorfer, I., Tschorner, I., Rogatsch, H., and Mikuz, G. (2004). Prognostic significance of tenascin-C expression in superficial and invasive bladder cancer. J Clin Pathol 57, 927-931.

Burchardt, E. R., Hein, R., and Bosserhoff, A. K. (2003). Laminin, hyaluronan, tenascin-C and type VI collagen levels in sera from patients with malignant melanoma. Clin Exp Dermatol 28, 515-520.

Burnett, J. C., and Rossi, J. J. (2012). RNA-based therapeutics: current progress and future prospects. Chem Biol 19, 60-71.

Cai, M., Onoda, K., Takao, M., Kyoko, I. Y., Shimpo, H., Yoshida, T., and Yada, I. (2002). Degradation of tenascin-C and activity of matrix metalloproteinase-2 are associated with tumor recurrence in early stage non-small cell lung cancer. Clin Cancer Res 8, 1152-1156.

Calvo, A., Catena, R., Noble, M. S., Carbott, D., Gil-Bazo, I., Gonzalez-Moreno, O., Huh, J. I., Sharp, R., Qiu, T. H., Anver, M. R., et al. (2008). Identification of VEGF-regulated genes associated with increased lung metastatic potential: functional involvement of tenascin-C in tumor growth and lung metastasis. Oncogene 27, 5373-5384.

Campbell, N. E., Kellenberger, L., Greenaway, J., Moorehead, R. A., Linnerth-Petrik, N. M., and Petrik, J. (2010). Extracellular matrix proteins and tumor angiogenesis. J Oncol 2010, 586905.

Canfield, A. E., and Schor, A. M. (1995). Evidence that tenascin and thrombospondin-1 modulate sprouting of endothelial cells. J Cell Sci 108 ( Pt 2), 797-809.

Carnemolla, B., Castellani, P., Ponassi, M., Borsi, L., Urbini, S., Nicolo, G., Dorcaratto, A., Viale, G., Winter, G., Neri, D., and Zardi, L. (1999). Identification of a glioblastoma-associated tenascin-C isoform by a high affinity recombinant antibody. Am J Pathol 154, 1345-1352.

Castellon, R., Caballero, S., Hamdi, H. K., Atilano, S. R., Aoki, A. M., Tarnuzzer, R. W., Kenney, M. C., Grant, M. B., and Ljubimov, A. V. (2002). Effects of tenascin-C on normal and diabetic retinal endothelial cells in culture. Invest Ophthalmol Vis Sci 43, 2758-2766.

Chambers, A. F., Groom, A. C., and MacDonald, I. C. (2002). Dissemination and growth of cancer cells in metastatic sites. Nat Rev Cancer 2, 563-572.

Chen, J., Chen, Z., Chen, M., Li, D., Li, Z., Xiong, Y., Dong, J., and Li, X. (2009). Role of fibrillar Tenascin-C in metastatic pancreatic cancer. Int J Oncol 34, 1029-1036.

Chi, A. S., Sorensen, A. G., Jain, R. K., and Batchelor, T. T. (2009). Angiogenesis as a therapeutic target in malignant gliomas. Oncologist 14, 621-636.

Chiquet, M., and Fambrough, D. M. (1984). Chick myotendinous antigen. II. A novel extracellular glycoprotein complex consisting of large disulfide-linked subunits. J Cell Biol 98, 1937-1946.

Chiquet-Ehrismann, R., Kalla, P., Pearson, C. A., Beck, K., and Chiquet, M. (1988). Tenascin interferes with fibronectin action. Cell 53, 383-390.

Chiquet-Ehrismann, R., Mackie, E. J., Pearson, C. A., and Sakakura, T. (1986). Tenascin: an extracellular matrix protein involved in tissue interactions during fetal development and oncogenesis. Cell *47*, 131-139.

Chiquet-Ehrismann, R., Matsuoka, Y., Hofer, U., Spring, J., Bernasconi, C., and Chiquet, M. (1991). Tenascin variants: differential binding to fibronectin and distinct distribution in cell cultures and tissues. Cell Regul *2*, 927-938.

Chiquet-Ehrismann, R., and Tucker, R. P. (2011). Tenascins and the importance of adhesion modulation. Cold Spring Harb Perspect Biol *3*.

Chung, C. Y., and Erickson, H. P. (1994). Cell surface annexin II is a high affinity receptor for the alternatively spliced segment of tenascin-C. J Cell Biol *126*, 539-548.

Chung, C. Y., and Erickson, H. P. (1997). Glycosaminoglycans modulate fibronectin matrix assembly and are essential for matrix incorporation of tenascin-C. J Cell Sci *110 ( Pt 12)*, 1413-1419.

Chung, C. Y., Murphy-Ullrich, J. E., and Erickson, H. P. (1996). Mitogenesis, cell migration, and loss of focal adhesions induced by tenascin-C interacting with its cell surface receptor, annexin II. Mol Biol Cell *7*, 883-892.

Chung, C. Y., Zardi, L., and Erickson, H. P. (1995). Binding of tenascin-C to soluble fibronectin and matrix fibrils. J Biol Chem *270*, 29012-29017.

Clark, R. A., Erickson, H. P., and Springer, T. A. (1997). Tenascin supports lymphocyte rolling. J Cell Biol *137*, 755-765.

Colman, H., Zhang, L., Sulman, E. P., McDonald, J. M., Shooshtari, N. L., Rivera, A., Popoff, S., Nutt, C. L., Louis, D. N., Cairncross, J. G., *et al.* (2010). A multigene predictor of outcome in glioblastoma. Neuro Oncol *12*, 49-57.

Coussens, L. M., Zitvogel, L., and Palucka, A. K. (2013). Neutralizing tumor-promoting chronic inflammation: a magic bullet? Science *339*, 286-291.

Czopka, T., von Holst, A., ffrench-Constant, C., and Faissner, A. (2010). Regulatory mechanisms that mediate tenascin C-dependent inhibition of oligodendrocyte precursor differentiation. J Neurosci *30*, 12310-12322.

Dandachi, N., Hauser-Kronberger, C., More, E., Wiesener, B., Hacker, G. W., Dietze, O., and Wirl, G. (2001). Co-expression of tenascin-C and vimentin in human breast cancer cells indicates phenotypic transdifferentiation during tumour progression: correlation with histopathological parameters, hormone receptors, and oncoproteins. J Pathol *193*, 181-189.

Daniels, D. A., Chen, H., Hicke, B. J., Swiderek, K. M., and Gold, L. (2003). A tenascin-C aptamer identified by tumor cell SELEX: systematic evolution of ligands by exponential enrichment. Proc Natl Acad Sci U S A *100*, 15416-15421.

Day, J. M., Olin, A. I., Murdoch, A. D., Canfield, A., Sasaki, T., Timpl, R., Hardingham, T. E., and Aspberg, A. (2004). Alternative splicing in the aggrecan G3 domain influences binding interactions with tenascin-C and other extracellular matrix proteins. J Biol Chem *279*, 12511-12518.

De Braud, F., Catania, C., Onofri, A., Pierantoni, C., Cascinu, S., Maur, M., Masini, C., Conte, P. F., Giovannoni, L., Tasciotti, A., *et al.* (2011). Combination of the immunocytokine F16-IL2 with doxorubicin or paclitaxel in patients with solid tumors: Results from two phase Ib trials. J Clin Oncol 29: ASCO Annual Meeting 2011 *Abstract 2595*.

De Laporte, L., Rice, J. J., Tortelli, F., and Hubbell, J. A. (2013). Tenascin C promiscuously binds growth factors via its fifth fibronectin type III-like domain. PLoS One *8*, e62076.

De Santis, R., Albertoni, C., Petronzelli, F., Campo, S., D'Alessio, V., Rosi, A., Anastasi, A. M., Lindstedt, R., Caroni, N., Arseni, B., *et al.* (2006). Low and high tenascin-expressing tumors are efficiently targeted by ST2146 monoclonal antibody. Clin Cancer Res *12*, 2191-2196.

De Wever, O., Nguyen, Q. D., Van Hoorde, L., Bracke, M., Bruyneel, E., Gespach, C., and Mareel, M. (2004). Tenascin-C and SF/HGF produced by myofibroblasts in vitro provide convergent pro-invasive signals to human colon cancer cells through RhoA and Rac. Faseb J *18*, 1016-1018.

Deen, S., and Ball, R. Y. (1994). Basement membrane and extracellular interstitial matrix components in bladder neoplasia--evidence of angiogenesis. Histopathology *25*, 475-481.

Dejana, E. (2010). The role of wnt signaling in physiological and pathological angiogenesis. Circ Res *107*, 943-952.

Delaney, C. E., Weagant, B. T., and Addison, C. L. (2006). The inhibitory effects of endostatin on endothelial cells are modulated by extracellular matrix. Exp Cell Res *312*, 2476-2489.

Denda, S., Muller, U., Crossin, K. L., Erickson, H. P., and Reichardt, L. F. (1998). Utilization of a soluble integrin-alkaline phosphatase chimera to characterize integrin alpha 8 beta 1 receptor interactions with tenascin: murine alpha 8 beta 1 binds to the RGD site in tenascin-C fragments, but not to native tenascin-C. Biochemistry *37*, 5464-5474.

Deryugina, E. I., and Bourdon, M. A. (1996). Tenascin mediates human glioma cell migration and modulates cell migration on fibronectin. J Cell Sci *109 ( Pt 3)*, 643-652.

Doi, D., Araki, T., and Asano, G. (1996). Immunohistochemical localization of tenascin, estrogen receptor and transforming growth factor-beta 1 in human endometrial carcinoma. Gynecol Obstet Invest *41*, 61-66.

Drumea-Mirancea, M., Wessels, J. T., Muller, C. A., Essl, M., Eble, J. A., Tolosa, E., Koch, M., Reinhardt, D. P., Sixt, M., Sorokin, L., *et al.* (2006). Characterization of a conduit system containing laminin-5 in the human thymus: a potential transport system for small molecules. J Cell Sci *119*, 1396-1405.

Dueck, M., Riedl, S., Hinz, U., Tandara, A., Moller, P., Herfarth, C., and Faissner, A. (1999). Detection of tenascin-C isoforms in colorectal mucosa, ulcerative colitis, carcinomas and liver metastases. Int J Cancer *82*, 477-483.

Dugu, L., Hayashida, S., Nakahara, T., Xie, L., Iwashita, Y., Liu, X., Uchi, H., Tateuchi, S., Takahara, M., Oda, Y., *et al.* (2010). Aberrant expression of tenascin-c and neuronatin in malignant peripheral nerve sheath tumors. Eur J Dermatol *20*, 580-584.

Dupont, S., Morsut, L., Aragona, M., Enzo, E., Giulitti, S., Cordenonsi, M., Zanconato, F., Le Digabel, J., Forcato, M., Bicciato, S., *et al.* (2011). Role of YAP/TAZ in mechanotransduction. Nature *474*, 179-183.

Ebos, J. M., Lee, C. R., Cruz-Munoz, W., Bjarnason, G. A., Christensen, J. G., and Kerbel, R. S. (2009). Accelerated metastasis after short-term treatment with a potent inhibitor of tumor angiogenesis. Cancer Cell *15*, 232-239.

El-Karef, A., Yoshida, T., Gabazza, E. C., Nishioka, T., Inada, H., Sakakura, T., and Imanaka-Yoshida, K. (2007). Deficiency of tenascin-C attenuates liver fibrosis in immune-mediated chronic hepatitis in mice. J Pathol *211*, 86-94.

Emoto, K., Yamada, Y., Sawada, H., Fujimoto, H., Ueno, M., Takayama, T., Kamada, K., Naito, A., Hirao, S., and Nakajima, Y. (2001). Annexin II overexpression correlates with stromal tenascin-C overexpression: a prognostic marker in colorectal carcinoma. Cancer *92*, 1419-1426.

Erickson, H. P., and Inglesias, J. L. (1984). A six-armed oligomer isolated from cell surface fibronectin preparations. Nature *311*, 267-269.

Erickson, H. P., and Taylor, H. C. (1987). Hexabrachion proteins in embryonic chicken tissues and human tumors. J Cell Biol *105*, 1387-1394.

Esposito, I., Penzel, R., Chaib-Harrireche, M., Barcena, U., Bergmann, F., Riedl, S., Kayed, H., Giese, N., Kleeff, J., Friess, H., and Schirmacher, P. (2006). Tenascin C and annexin II expression in the process of pancreatic carcinogenesis. J Pathol *208*, 673-685.

Faissner, A., Kruse, J., Kuhn, K., and Schachner, M. (1990). Binding of the J1 adhesion molecules to extracellular matrix constituents. J Neurochem *54*, 1004-1015.

Fantozzi, A., and Christofori, G. (2006). Mouse models of breast cancer metastasis. Breast Cancer Res *8*, 212.

Felix, A., Rosa, J. C., Fonseca, I., Cidadao, A., and Soares, J. (2004). Pleomorphic adenoma and carcinoma ex pleomorphic adenoma: immunohistochemical demonstration of the association between tenascin expression and malignancy. Histopathology *45*, 187-192.

Felix, A., Rosa, J. C., Nunes, J. F., Fonseca, I., Cidadao, A., and Soares, J. (2002). Hyalinizing clear cell carcinoma of salivary glands: a study of extracellular matrix. Oral Oncol *38*, 364-368.

Ferguson, J. E., Schor, A. M., Howell, A., and Ferguson, M. W. (1990). Tenascin distribution in the normal human breast is altered during the menstrual cycle and in carcinoma. Differentiation *42*, 199-207.

Fischer, D., Chiquet-Ehrismann, R., Bernasconi, C., and Chiquet, M. (1995). A single heparin binding region within the fibrinogen-like domain is functional in chick tenascin-C. J Biol Chem *270*, 3378-3384.

Forsberg, E., Hirsch, E., Frohlich, L., Meyer, M., Ekblom, P., Aszodi, A., Werner, S., and Fassler, R. (1996). Skin wounds and severed nerves heal normally in mice lacking tenascin-C. Proc Natl Acad Sci U S A *93*, 6594-6599.

Fouda, G. G., Jaeger, F. H., Amos, J. D., Ho, C., Kunz, E. L., Anasti, K., Stamper, L. W., Liebl, B. E., Barbas, K. H., Ohashi, T., *et al.* (2013). Tenascin-C is an innate broad-spectrum, HIV-1-neutralizing protein in breast milk. Proc Natl Acad Sci U S A *110*, 18220-18225.

Franchi, A., and Santucci, M. (1996). Tenascin expression in cutaneous fibrohistiocytic tumors. Immunohistochemical investigation of 24 cases. Am J Dermatopathol *18*, 454-459.

Frey, K., Fiechter, M., Schwager, K., Belloni, B., Barysch, M. J., Neri, D., and Dummer, R. (2011). Different patterns of fibronectin and tenascin-C splice variants expression in primary and metastatic melanoma lesions. Exp Dermatol *20*, 685-688.

Friedman, H. S., Prados, M. D., Wen, P. Y., Mikkelsen, T., Schiff, D., Abrey, L. E., Yung, W. K., Paleologos, N., Nicholas, M. K., Jensen, R., *et al.* (2009). Bevacizumab alone and in combination with irinotecan in recurrent glioblastoma. J Clin Oncol *27*, 4733-4740.

Fukunaga-Kalabis, M., Martinez, G., Nguyen, T. K., Kim, D., Santiago-Walker, A., Roesch, A., and Herlyn, M. (2010). Tenascin-C promotes melanoma progression by maintaining the ABCB5-positive side population. Oncogene *29*, 6115-6124.

Gaggioli, C., Hooper, S., Hidalgo-Carcedo, C., Grosse, R., Marshall, J. F., Harrington, K., and Sahai, E. (2007). Fibroblast-led collective invasion of carcinoma cells with differing roles for RhoGTPases in leading and following cells. Nat Cell Biol *9*, 1392-1400.

Galler, K., Junker, K., Franz, M., Hentschel, J., Richter, P., Gajda, M., Gohlert, A., von Eggeling, F., Heller, R., Giavazzi, R., *et al.* (2012). Differential vascular expression and regulation of oncofetal tenascin-C and fibronectin variants in renal cell carcinoma (RCC): implications for an individualized angiogenesis-related targeted drug delivery. Histochem Cell Biol *137*, 195-204.

Galoian, K. A., Garamszegi, N., Garamszegi, S. P., and Scully, S. P. (2007). Molecular mechanism of tenascin-C action on matrix metalloproteinase-1 invasive potential. Exp Biol Med (Maywood) 232, 515-522.

Garcion, E., Faissner, A., and ffrench-Constant, C. (2001). Knockout mice reveal a contribution of the extracellular matrix molecule tenascin-C to neural precursor proliferation and migration. Development 128, 2485-2496.

Garcion, E., Halilagic, A., Faissner, A., and ffrench-Constant, C. (2004). Generation of an environmental niche for neural stem cell development by the extracellular matrix molecule tenascin C. Development 131, 3423-3432.

Gardner, T., Elzey, B., and Hahn, N. M. (2012). Sipuleucel-T (Provenge) autologous vaccine approved for treatment of men with asymptomatic or minimally symptomatic castrate-resistant metastatic prostate cancer. Hum Vaccin Immunother 8, 534-539.

Gazzaniga, P., Nofroni, I., Gandini, O., Silvestri, I., Frati, L., Agliano, A. M., and Gradilone, A. (2005). Tenascin C and epidermal growth factor receptor as markers of circulating tumoral cells in bladder and colon cancer. Oncol Rep 14, 1199-1202.

Germano, A., Galatioto, S., Caffo, M., Caruso, G., La Torre, D., Cardia, E., and Tomasello, F. (2000). Immunohistochemical tenascin-C expression in paediatric supratentorial glioblastoma multiforme. Childs Nerv Syst 16, 357-362.

Ghert, M. A., Jung, S. T., Qi, W., Harrelson, J. M., Erickson, H. P., Block, J. A., and Scully, S. P. (2001). The clinical significance of tenascin-C splice variant expression in chondrosarcoma. Oncology 61, 306-314.

Gherzi, R., Ponassi, M., Gaggero, B., and Zardi, L. (1995). The first untranslated exon of the human tenascin-C gene plays a regulatory role in gene transcription. FEBS Lett 369, 335-339.

Goepel, C., Buchmann, J., Schultka, R., and Koelbl, H. (2000). Tenascin-A marker for the malignant potential of preinvasive breast cancers. Gynecol Oncol 79, 372-378.

Goepel, C., Stoerer, S., and Koelbl, H. (2003). Tenascin in preinvasive lesions of the vulva and vulvar cancer. Anticancer Res 23, 4587-4591.

Goh, F. G., Piccinini, A. M., Krausgruber, T., Udalova, I. A., and Midwood, K. S. (2010). Transcriptional regulation of the endogenous danger signal tenascin-C: a novel autocrine loop in inflammation. J Immunol *184*, 2655-2662.

Gong, X. G., Lv, Y. F., Li, X. Q., Xu, F. G., and Ma, Q. Y. (2010). Gemcitabine resistance induced by interaction between alternatively spliced segment of tenascin-C and annexin A2 in pancreatic cancer cells. Biol Pharm Bull *33*, 1261-1267.

Gotz, M., Stoykova, A., and Gruss, P. (1998). Pax6 controls radial glia differentiation in the cerebral cortex. Neuron *21*, 1031-1044.

Gould, V. E., Koukoulis, G. K., and Virtanen, I. (1990). Extracellular matrix proteins and their receptors in the normal, hyperplastic and neoplastic breast. Cell Differ Dev *32*, 409-416.

Goussia, A. C., Ioachim, E. E., Peschos, D., Assimakopoulos, D. A., Skevas, A., and Agnantis, N. J. (2000). Expression of the extracellular matrix protein tenascin in laryngeal epithelial lesions: correlation with fibronectin, CD44, cathepsin D and proliferation indices. Virchows Arch *436*, 579-584.

Grahovac, J., Becker, D., and Wells, A. (2012). Melanoma Cell Invasiveness Is Promoted at Least in Part by the Epidermal Growth Factor-Like Repeats of Tenascin-C. J Invest Dermatol.

Grumet, M., Hoffman, S., Crossin, K. L., and Edelman, G. M. (1985). Cytotactin, an extracellular matrix protein of neural and non-neural tissues that mediates glia-neuron interaction. Proc Natl Acad Sci U S A *82*, 8075-8079.

Gutbrodt, K. L., Schliemann, C., Giovannoni, L., Frey, K., Pabst, T., Klapper, W., Berdel, W. E., and Neri, D. (2013). Antibody-based delivery of interleukin-2 to neovasculature has potent activity against acute myeloid leukemia. Sci Transl Med *5*, 201ra118.

Guttery, D. S., Hancox, R. A., Mulligan, K. T., Hughes, S., Lambe, S. M., Pringle, J. H., Walker, R. A., Jones, J. L., and Shaw, J. A. (2010a). Association of invasion-promoting tenascin-C additional domains with breast cancers in young women. Breast Cancer Res *12*, R57.

Guttery, D. S., Shaw, J. A., Lloyd, K., Pringle, J. H., and Walker, R. A. (2010b). Expression of tenascin-C and its isoforms in the breast. Cancer Metastasis Rev *29*, 595-606.

Hagedorn, H., Sauer, U., Schleicher, E., and Nerlich, A. (1999). Expression of TGF-beta 1 protein and mRNA and the effect on the tissue remodeling in laryngeal carcinomas. Anticancer Res *19*, 4265-4272.

Halder, G., Dupont, S., and Piccolo, S. (2012). Transduction of mechanical and cytoskeletal cues by YAP and TAZ. Nature reviews Molecular cell biology *13*, 591-600.

Han, J. Y., Kim, H. S., Lee, S. H., Park, W. S., Lee, J. Y., and Yoo, N. J. (2003). Immunohistochemical expression of integrins and extracellular matrix proteins in non-small cell lung cancer: correlation with lymph node metastasis. Lung Cancer *41*, 65-70.

Hanahan, D. (1985). Heritable formation of pancreatic beta-cell tumours in transgenic mice expressing recombinant insulin/simian virus 40 oncogenes. Nature *315*, 115-122.

Hanahan, D., and Weinberg, R. A. (2011). Hallmarks of cancer: the next generation. Cell *144*, 646-674.

Hanamura, N., Yoshida, T., Matsumoto, E., Kawarada, Y., and Sakakura, T. (1997). Expression of fibronectin and tenascin-C mRNA by myofibroblasts, vascular cells and epithelial cells in human colon adenomas and carcinomas. Int J Cancer *73*, 10-15.

Hancox, R. A., Allen, M. D., Holliday, D. L., Edwards, D. R., Pennington, C. J., Guttery, D. S., Shaw, J. A., Walker, R. A., Pringle, J. H., and Jones, J. L. (2009). Tumour-associated tenascin-C isoforms promote breast cancer cell invasion and growth by matrix metalloproteinase-dependent and independent mechanisms. Breast Cancer Res *11*, R24.

Helleman, J., Jansen, M. P., Ruigrok-Ritstier, K., van Staveren, I. L., Look, M. P., Meijer-van Gelder, M. E., Sieuwerts, A. M., Klijn, J. G., Sleijfer, S., Foekens, J. A., and Berns, E. M. (2008). Association of an extracellular matrix gene cluster with breast cancer prognosis and endocrine therapy response. Clin Cancer Res *14*, 5555-5564.

Herold-Mende, C., Mueller, M. M., Bonsanto, M. M., Schmitt, H. P., Kunze, S., and Steiner, H. H. (2002). Clinical impact and functional aspects of tenascin-C expression during glioma progression. Int J Cancer *98*, 362-369.

Heuveling, D. A., de Bree, R., Vugts, D. J., Huisman, M. C., Giovannoni, L., Hoekstra, O. S., Leemans, C. R., Neri, D., and van Dongen, G. A. (2013). Phase 0 microdosing PET study using the human mini antibody F16SIP in head and neck cancer patients. J Nucl Med *54*, 397-401.

Hicke, B. J., Marion, C., Chang, Y. F., Gould, T., Lynott, C. K., Parma, D., Schmidt, P. G., and Warren, S. (2001). Tenascin-C aptamers are generated using tumor cells and purified protein. J Biol Chem *276*, 48644-48654.

Hicke, B. J., Stephens, A. W., Gould, T., Chang, Y. F., Lynott, C. K., Heil, J., Borkowski, S., Hilger, C. S., Cook, G., Warren, S., and Schmidt, P. G. (2006). Tumor targeting by an aptamer. J Nucl Med *47*, 668-678.

Higuchi, M., Ohnishi, T., Arita, N., Hiraga, S., and Hayakawa, T. (1993). Expression of tenascin in human gliomas: its relation to histological malignancy, tumor dedifferentiation and angiogenesis. Acta Neuropathol *85*, 481-487.

Hill, J. J., Tremblay, T. L., Pen, A., Li, J., Robotham, A. C., Lenferink, A. E., Wang, E., O'Connor-McCourt, M., and Kelly, J. F. (2011). Identification of vascular breast tumor markers by laser capture microdissection and label-free LC-MS. J Proteome Res *10*, 2479-2493.

Hindermann, W., Berndt, A., Borsi, L., Luo, X., Hyckel, P., Katenkamp, D., and Kosmehl, H. (1999). Synthesis and protein distribution of the unspliced large tenascin-C isoform in oral squamous cell carcinoma. J Pathol *189*, 475-480.

Hirata, E., Arakawa, Y., Shirahata, M., Yamaguchi, M., Kishi, Y., Okada, T., Takahashi, J. A., Matsuda, M., and Hashimoto, N. (2009). Endogenous tenascin-C enhances glioblastoma invasion with reactive change of surrounding brain tissue. Cancer Sci *100*, 1451-1459.

Huang, J. Y., Cheng, Y. J., Lin, Y. P., Lin, H. C., Su, C. C., Juliano, R., and Yang, B. C. (2010). Extracellular matrix of glioblastoma inhibits polarization and transmigration of T cells: the role of tenascin-C in immune suppression. J Immunol *185*, 1450-1459.

Huang, W., Chiquet-Ehrismann, R., Moyano, J. V., Garcia-Pardo, A., and Orend, G. (2001). Interference of tenascin-C with syndecan-4 binding to fibronectin blocks cell adhesion and stimulates tumor cell proliferation. Cancer Res *61*, 8586-8594.

Huber, M. A., Kraut, N., and Beug, H. (2005). Molecular requirements for epithelial-mesenchymal transition during tumor progression. Curr Opin Cell Biol 17, 548-558.

Huijbers, E. J. (2012) Development of a Cancer Vaccine Targeting Tumor Blood Vessels, Uppsala Universitet, Uppsala; http://urn.kb.se/resolve?urn=urn:nbn:se:uu:diva-170887.

Huijbers, E. J., Ringvall, M., Femel, J., Kalamajski, S., Lukinius, A., Abrink, M., Hellman, L., and Olsson, A. K. (2010). Vaccination against the extra domain-B of fibronectin as a novel tumor therapy. Faseb J 24, 4535-4544.

Hynes, R. O. (2009). The extracellular matrix: not just pretty fibrils. Science 326, 1216-1219.

IACR (2008). International Agency for Research on Cancer, http://globocan.iarc.fr.

Ide, M., Saito, K., Tsutsumi, S., Tsuboi, K., Yamaguchi, S., Asao, T., Kuwano, H., and Nakajima, T. (2007). Over-expression of 14-3-3sigma in budding colorectal cancer cells modulates cell migration in the presence of tenascin-C. Oncol Rep 18, 1451-1456.

Ikeda, Y., Mori, M., Kajiyama, K., Haraguchi, Y., Sasaki, O., and Sugimachi, K. (1995). Immunohistochemical expression of tenascin in normal stomach tissue, gastric carcinomas and gastric carcinoma in lymph nodes. Br J Cancer 72, 189-192.

Ilmonen, S., Jahkola, T., Turunen, J. P., Muhonen, T., and Asko-Seljavaara, S. (2004). Tenascin-C in primary malignant melanoma of the skin. Histopathology 45, 405-411.

Ilunga, K., and Iriyama, K. (1995). Expression of tenascin in gastric carcinoma. Br J Surg 82, 948-951.

Ilunga, K., Nishiura, R., Inada, H., El-Karef, A., Imanaka-Yoshida, K., Sakakura, T., and Yoshida, T. (2004). Co-stimulation of human breast cancer cells with transforming growth factor-beta and tenascin-C enhances matrix metalloproteinase-9 expression and cancer cell invasion. Int J Exp Pathol 85, 373-379.

Ingham, K. C., Brew, S. A., and Erickson, H. P. (2004). Localization of a cryptic binding site for tenascin on fibronectin. J Biol Chem 279, 28132-28135.

Ioachim, E., Charchanti, A., Briasoulis, E., Karavasilis, V., Tsanou, H., Arvanitis, D. L., Agnantis, N. J., and Pavlidis, N. (2002). Immunohistochemical expression of extracellular matrix components tenascin, fibronectin, collagen type IV and laminin in breast cancer: their prognostic value and role in tumour invasion and progression. Eur J Cancer *38*, 2362-2370.

Ioachim, E., Michael, M., Stavropoulos, N. E., Kitsiou, E., Salmas, M., and Malamou-Mitsi, V. (2005). A clinicopathological study of the expression of extracellular matrix components in urothelial carcinoma. BJU Int *95*, 655-659.

Ishihara, A., Yoshida, T., Tamaki, H., and Sakakura, T. (1995). Tenascin expression in cancer cells and stroma of human breast cancer and its prognostic significance. Clin Cancer Res *1*, 1035-1041.

Ishii, S., Ohbu, M., Toomine, Y., Nishimura, Y., Hattori, M., Yokoyama, M., Toyonaga, M., Kakinuma, H., and Matsumoto, K. (2011). Immunohistochemical, molecular, and clinicopathological analyses of urothelial carcinoma, micropapillary variant. Pathol Int *61*, 723-730.

Ishitsuka, T., Ikuta, T., Ariga, H., and Matsumoto, K. (2009). Serum tenascin-X strongly binds to vascular endothelial growth factor. Biol Pharm Bull *32*, 1004-1011.

Ishiwata, T., Takahashi, K., Shimanuki, Y., Ohashi, R., Cui, R., Takahashi, F., Shimizu, K., Miura, K., and Fukuchi, Y. (2005). Serum tenascin-C as a potential predictive marker of angiogenesis in non-small cell lung cancer. Anticancer Res *25*, 489-495.

Iskaros, B. F., Hu, X., Sparano, J. A., and Fineberg, S. A. (1998). Tenascin pattern of expression and established prognostic factors in invasive breast carcinoma. J Surg Oncol *68*, 107-112.

Iskaros, B. F., Tanaka, K. E., Hu, X., Kadish, A. S., and Steinberg, J. J. (1997). Morphologic pattern of tenascin as a diagnostic biomarker in colon cancer. J Surg Oncol *64*, 98-101.

Itoh, M., Haga, I., Li, Q. H., and Fujisawa, J. (2002). Identification of cellular mRNA targets for RNA-binding protein Sam68. Nucleic Acids Res *30*, 5452-5464.

Jahkola, T., Toivonen, T., Nordling, S., von Smitten, K., and Virtanen, I. (1998a). Expression of tenascin-C in intraductal carcinoma of human breast: relationship to invasion. Eur J Cancer 34, 1687-1692.

Jahkola, T., Toivonen, T., Virtanen, I., von Smitten, K., Nordling, S., von Boguslawski, K., Haglund, C., Nevanlinna, H., and Blomqvist, C. (1998b). Tenascin-C expression in invasion border of early breast cancer: a predictor of local and distant recurrence. Br J Cancer 78, 1507-1513.

Jahkola, T., Toivonen, T., von Smitten, K., Blomqvist, C., and Virtanen, I. (1996). Expression of tenascin in invasion border of early breast cancer correlates with higher risk of distant metastasis. Int J Cancer 69, 445-447.

Jang, J. H., Hwang, J. H., Chung, C. P., and Choung, P. H. (2004). Identification and kinetics analysis of a novel heparin-binding site (KEDK) in human tenascin-C. J Biol Chem 279, 25562-25566.

Jones, F. S., Hoffman, S., Cunningham, B. A., and Edelman, G. M. (1989). A detailed structural model of cytotactin: protein homologies, alternative RNA splicing, and binding regions. Proc Natl Acad Sci U S A 86, 1905-1909.

Joshi, P., Chung, C. Y., Aukhil, I., and Erickson, H. P. (1993). Endothelial cells adhere to the RGD domain and the fibrinogen-like terminal knob of tenascin. J Cell Sci 106 ( Pt 1), 389-400.

Juhasz, A., Bardos, H., Repassy, G., and Adany, R. (2000). Characteristic distribution patterns of tenascin in laryngeal and hypopharyngeal cancers. Laryngoscope 110, 84-92.

Juuti, A., Nordling, S., Louhimo, J., Lundin, J., and Haglund, C. (2004). Tenascin C expression is upregulated in pancreatic cancer and correlates with differentiation. J Clin Pathol 57, 1151-1155.

Kaariainen, E., Nummela, P., Soikkeli, J., Yin, M., Lukk, M., Jahkola, T., Virolainen, S., Ora, A., Ukkonen, E., Saksela, O., and Holtta, E. (2006). Switch to an invasive growth phase in melanoma is associated with tenascin-C, fibronectin, and procollagen-I forming specific channel structures for invasion. J Pathol 210, 181-191.

Kaarteenaho-Wiik, R., Soini, Y., Pollanen, R., Paakko, P., and Kinnula, V. L. (2003). Over-expression of tenascin-C in malignant pleural mesothelioma. Histopathology 42, 280-291.

Kahn, N., Meister, M., Eberhardt, R., Muley, T., Schnabel, P. A., Bender, C., Johannes, M., Keitel, D., Sultmann, H., Herth, F. J., and Kuner, R. (2012). Early detection of lung cancer by molecular markers in endobronchial epithelial-lining fluid. J Thorac Oncol 7, 1001-1008.

Kammerer, R. A., Schulthess, T., Landwehr, R., Lustig, A., Fischer, D., and Engel, J. (1998). Tenascin-C hexabrachion assembly is a sequential two-step process initiated by coiled-coil alpha-helices. J Biol Chem 273, 10602-10608.

Kanayama, M., Kurotaki, D., Morimoto, J., Asano, T., Matsui, Y., Nakayama, Y., Saito, Y., Ito, K., Kimura, C., Iwasaki, N., et al. (2009). Alpha9 integrin and its ligands constitute critical joint microenvironments for development of autoimmune arthritis. J Immunol 182, 8015-8025.

Kanayama, M., Morimoto, J., Matsui, Y., Ikesue, M., Danzaki, K., Kurotaki, D., Ito, K., Yoshida, T., and Uede, T. (2011). alpha9beta1 integrin-mediated signaling serves as an intrinsic regulator of pathogenic Th17 cell generation. J Immunol 187, 5851-5864.

Kang, Y., Siegel, P. M., Shu, W., Drobnjak, M., Kakonen, S. M., Cordon-Cardo, C., Guise, T. A., and Massague, J. (2003). A multigenic program mediating breast cancer metastasis to bone. Cancer Cell 3, 537-549.

Karja, V., Syrjanen, K., and Syrjanen, S. (1995). Collagen IV and tenascin immunoreactivity as prognostic determinant in benign and malignant salivary gland tumours. Acta Otolaryngol 115, 569-575.

Katenkamp, K., Berndt, A., Hindermann, W., Wunderlich, H., Haas, K. M., Borsi, L., Zardi, L., and Kosmehl, H. (2004). mRNA expression and protein distribution of the unspliced tenascin-C isoform in prostatic adenocarcinoma. J Pathol 203, 771-779.

Katoh, D., Nagaharu, K., Shimojo, N., Hanamura, N., Yamashita, M., Kozuka, Y., Imanaka-Yoshida, K., and Yoshida, T. (2013). Binding of alphavbeta1 and alphavbeta6 integrins to tenascin-C induces epithelial-mesenchymal transition-like change of breast cancer cells. Oncogenesis 2, e65.

Kii, I., Nishiyama, T., Li, M., Matsumoto, K., Saito, M., Amizuka, N., and Kudo, A. (2010). Incorporation of tenascin-C into the extracellular matrix by periostin underlies an extracellular meshwork architecture. J Biol Chem *285*, 2028-2039.

Kim, K., Lu, Z., and Hay, E. D. (2002). Direct evidence for a role of beta-catenin/LEF-1 signaling pathway in induction of EMT. Cell Biol Int *26*, 463-476.

Klein, G., Beck, S., and Muller, C. A. (1993). Tenascin is a cytoadhesive extracellular matrix component of the human hematopoietic microenvironment. J Cell Biol *123*, 1027-1035.

Ko, H. Y., Choi, K. J., Lee, C. H., and Kim, S. (2011). A multimodal nanoparticle-based cancer imaging probe simultaneously targeting nucleolin, integrin alphavbeta3 and tenascin-C proteins. Biomaterials *32*, 1130-1138.

Koljonen, V., Jahkola, T., Tukiainen, E., Granroth, G., Haglund, C., and Bohling, T. (2005). Tenascin-C in primary Merkel cell carcinoma. J Clin Pathol *58*, 297-300.

Korshunov, A., Golanov, A., Ozerov, S., and Sycheva, R. (1999). Prognostic value of tumor-associated antigens immunoreactivity and apoptosis in medulloblastomas. An analysis of 73 cases. Brain Tumor Pathol *16*, 37-44.

Korshunov, A., Golanov, A., and Timirgaz, V. (2000). Immunohistochemical markers for intracranial ependymoma recurrence. An analysis of 88 cases. J Neurol Sci *177*, 72-82.

Kreisl, T. N., Kim, L., Moore, K., Duic, P., Royce, C., Stroud, I., Garren, N., Mackey, M., Butman, J. A., Camphausen, K., *et al.* (2009). Phase II trial of single-agent bevacizumab followed by bevacizumab plus irinotecan at tumor progression in recurrent glioblastoma. J Clin Oncol *27*, 740-745.

Kuhn, C., and Mason, R. J. (1995). Immunolocalization of SPARC, tenascin, and thrombospondin in pulmonary fibrosis. Am J Pathol *147*, 1759-1769.

Kuivanen, T., Tanskanen, M., Jahkola, T., Impola, U., Asko-Seljavaara, S., and Saarialho-Kere, U. (2004). Matrilysin-1 (MMP-7) and MMP-19 are expressed by Paget's cells in extramammary Paget's disease. J Cutan Pathol *31*, 483-491.

Kulla, A., Liigant, A., Piirsoo, A., Rippin, G., and Asser, T. (2000). Tenascin expression patterns and cells of monocyte lineage: relationship in human gliomas. Mod Pathol 13, 56-67.

Kuperwasser, C., Dessain, S., Bierbaum, B. E., Garnet, D., Sperandio, K., Gauvin, G. P., Naber, S. P., Weinberg, R. A., and Rosenblatt, M. (2005). A mouse model of human breast cancer metastasis to human bone. Cancer Res 65, 6130-6138.

Kusagawa, H., Onoda, K., Namikawa, S., Yada, I., Okada, A., Yoshida, T., and Sakakura, T. (1998). Expression and degeneration of tenascin-C in human lung cancers. Br J Cancer 77, 98-102.

Kuznetsova, S. A., and Roberts, D. D. (2004). Functional regulation of T lymphocytes by modulatory extracellular matrix proteins. Int J Biochem Cell Biol 36, 1126-1134.

Landemaine, T., Jackson, A., Bellahcene, A., Rucci, N., Sin, S., Abad, B. M., Sierra, A., Boudinet, A., Guinebretiere, J. M., Ricevuto, E., et al. (2008). A six-gene signature predicting breast cancer lung metastasis. Cancer Res 68, 6092-6099.

Lange, K., Kammerer, M., Hegi, M. E., Grotegut, S., Dittmann, A., Huang, W., Fluri, E., Yip, G. W., Gotte, M., Ruiz, C., and Orend, G. (2007). Endothelin receptor type B counteracts tenascin-C-induced endothelin receptor type A-dependent focal adhesion and actin stress fiber disorganization. Cancer Res 67, 6163-6173.

Lange, K., Kammerer, M., Saupe, F., Hegi, M. E., Grotegut, S., Fluri, E., and Orend, G. (2008). Combined lysophosphatidic acid/platelet-derived growth factor signaling triggers glioma cell migration in a tenascin-C microenvironment. Cancer Res 68, 6942-6952.

Lee, Y., Bullard, D. E., Humphrey, P. A., Colapinto, E. V., Friedman, H. S., Zalutsky, M. R., Coleman, R. E., and Bigner, D. D. (1988a). Treatment of intracranial human glioma xenografts with 131I-labeled anti-tenascin monoclonal antibody 81C6. Cancer Res 48, 2904-2910.

Lee, Y. S., Bullard, D. E., Zalutsky, M. R., Coleman, R. E., Wikstrand, C. J., Friedman, H. S., Colapinto, E. V., and Bigner, D. D. (1988b). Therapeutic efficacy of antiglioma mesenchymal extracellular matrix 131I-radiolabeled murine monoclonal antibody in a human glioma xenograft model. Cancer Res 48, 559-566.

Leins, A., Riva, P., Lindstedt, R., Davidoff, M. S., Mehraein, P., and Weis, S. (2003). Expression of tenascin-C in various human brain tumors and its relevance for survival in patients with astrocytoma. Cancer 98, 2430-2439.

Levental, K. R., Yu, H., Kass, L., Lakins, J. N., Egeblad, M., Erler, J. T., Fong, S. F., Csiszar, K., Giaccia, A., Weninger, W., et al. (2009). Matrix crosslinking forces tumor progression by enhancing integrin signaling. Cell 139, 891-906.

Lichtenberger, B. M., Tan, P. K., Niederleithner, H., Ferrara, N., Petzelbauer, P., and Sibilia, M. (2010). Autocrine VEGF signaling synergizes with EGFR in tumor cells to promote epithelial cancer development. Cell 140, 268-279.

Lightner, V. A., Marks, J. R., and McCachren, S. S. (1994). Epithelial cells are an important source of tenascin in normal and malignant human breast tissue. Exp Cell Res 210, 177-184.

Lillien, L., and Raphael, H. (2000). BMP and FGF regulate the development of EGF-responsive neural progenitor cells. Development 127, 4993-5005.

Linder, S., Castanos-Velez, E., von Rosen, A., and Biberfeld, P. (2001). Immunohistochemical expression of extracellular matrix proteins and adhesion molecules in pancreatic carcinoma. Hepatogastroenterology 48, 1321-1327.

Liu, R., He, Y., Li, B., Liu, J., Ren, Y., Han, W., Wang, X., and Zhang, L. (2012). Tenascin-C produced by oxidized LDL-stimulated macrophages increases foam cell formation through Toll-like receptor-4. Mol Cells 34, 35-41.

Loike, J. D., Cao, L., Budhu, S., Hoffman, S., and Silverstein, S. C. (2001). Blockade of alpha 5 beta 1 integrins reverses the inhibitory effect of tenascin on chemotaxis of human monocytes and polymorphonuclear leukocytes through three-dimensional gels of extracellular matrix proteins. J Immunol 166, 7534-7542.

Lu, P., Weaver, V. M., and Werb, Z. (2012). The extracellular matrix: a dynamic niche in cancer progression. J Cell Biol 196, 395-406.

Luczak, J. A., Redick, S. D., and Schwarzbauer, J. E. (1998). A single cysteine, Cys-64, is essential for assembly of tenascin-C hexabrachions. J Biol Chem 273, 2073-2077.

Lyons, A. J., and Jones, J. (2007). Cell adhesion molecules, the extracellular matrix and oral squamous carcinoma. Int J Oral Maxillofac Surg *36*, 671-679.

Mackie, E. J., Chiquet-Ehrismann, R., Pearson, C. A., Inaguma, Y., Taya, K., Kawarada, Y., and Sakakura, T. (1987). Tenascin is a stromal marker for epithelial malignancy in the mammary gland. Proc Natl Acad Sci U S A *84*, 4621-4625.

Mackie, E. J., and Tucker, R. P. (1999). The tenascin-C knockout revisited. J Cell Sci *112 ( Pt 22)*, 3847-3853.

Malanchi, I., Santamaria-Martinez, A., Susanto, E., Peng, H., Lehr, H. A., Delaloye, J. F., and Huelsken, J. (2011). Interactions between cancer stem cells and their niche govern metastatic colonization. Nature *481*, 85-89.

Mancuso, M. R., Davis, R., Norberg, S. M., O'Brien, S., Sennino, B., Nakahara, T., Yao, V. J., Inai, T., Brooks, P., Freimark, B., *et al.* (2006). Rapid vascular regrowth in tumors after reversal of VEGF inhibition. J Clin Invest *116*, 2610-2621.

Maniotis, A. J., Folberg, R., Hess, A., Seftor, E. A., Gardner, L. M., Pe'er, J., Trent, J. M., Meltzer, P. S., and Hendrix, M. J. (1999). Vascular channel formation by human melanoma cells in vivo and in vitro: vasculogenic mimicry. Am J Pathol *155*, 739-752.

Marlind, J., Kaspar, M., Trachsel, E., Sommavilla, R., Hindle, S., Bacci, C., Giovannoni, L., and Neri, D. (2008). Antibody-mediated delivery of interleukin-2 to the stroma of breast cancer strongly enhances the potency of chemotherapy. Clin Cancer Res *14*, 6515-6524.

Martin, D., Brown-Luedi, M., and Chiquet-Ehrismann, R. (2003). Tenascin-C signaling through induction of 14-3-3 tau. J Cell Biol *160*, 171-175.

Martina, E., Degen, M., Ruegg, C., Merlo, A., Lino, M. M., Chiquet-Ehrismann, R., and Brellier, F. (2010). Tenascin-W is a specific marker of glioma-associated blood vessels and stimulates angiogenesis in vitro. Faseb J *24*, 778-787.

Medzhitov, R., and Janeway, C. A., Jr. (2002). Decoding the patterns of self and nonself by the innate immune system. Science *296*, 298-300.

Melis, M., Baiocchini, A., Soda, G., and Bosco, D. (1997). Tenascin expression in elastotic cuffs of invasive ductal carcinoma of the breast. Pathol Res Pract *193*, 479-484.

Mercado, M. L., Nur-e-Kamal, A., Liu, H. Y., Gross, S. R., Movahed, R., and Meiners, S. (2004). Neurite outgrowth by the alternatively spliced region of human tenascin-C is mediated by neuronal alpha7beta1 integrin. J Neurosci *24*, 238-247.

Midwood, K., Sacre, S., Piccinini, A. M., Inglis, J., Trebaul, A., Chan, E., Drexler, S., Sofat, N., Kashiwagi, M., Orend, G., *et al.* (2009). Tenascin-C is an endogenous activator of Toll-like receptor 4 that is essential for maintaining inflammation in arthritic joint disease. Nat Med *15*, 774-780.

Midwood, K. S., Hussenet, T., Langlois, B., and Orend, G. (2011). Advances in tenascin-C biology. Cell Mol Life Sci *68*, 3175-3199.

Midwood, K. S., and Orend, G. (2009). The role of tenascin-C in tissue injury and tumorigenesis. J Cell Commun Signal *3*, 287-310.

Midwood, K. S., and Schwarzbauer, J. E. (2002). Tenascin-C modulates matrix contraction via focal adhesion kinase- and Rho-mediated signaling pathways. Mol Biol Cell *13*, 3601-3613.

Midwood, K. S., Valenick, L. V., Hsia, H. C., and Schwarzbauer, J. E. (2004a). Coregulation of fibronectin signaling and matrix contraction by tenascin-C and syndecan-4. Mol Biol Cell *15*, 5670-5677.

Midwood, K. S., Williams, L. V., and Schwarzbauer, J. E. (2004b). Tissue repair and the dynamics of the extracellular matrix. Int J Biochem Cell Biol *36*, 1031-1037.

Mighell, A. J., Thompson, J., Hume, W. J., Markham, A. F., and Robinson, P. A. (1997). Human tenascin-C: identification of a novel type III repeat in oral cancer and of novel splice variants in normal, malignant and reactive oral mucosae. Int J Cancer *72*, 236-240.

Milev, P., Fischer, D., Haring, M., Schulthess, T., Margolis, R. K., Chiquet-Ehrismann, R., and Margolis, R. U. (1997). The fibrinogen-like globe of tenascin-C mediates its interactions with neurocan and phosphacan/protein-tyrosine phosphatase-zeta/beta. J Biol Chem *272*, 15501-15509.

Min, J. K., Park, H., Choi, H. J., Kim, Y., Pyun, B. J., Agrawal, V., Song, B. W., Jeon, J., Maeng, Y. S., Rho, S. S., *et al.* (2011). The WNT antagonist Dickkopf2 promotes angiogenesis in rodent and human endothelial cells. J Clin Invest *121*, 1882-1893.

Minn, A. J., Gupta, G. P., Siegel, P. M., Bos, P. D., Shu, W., Giri, D. D., Viale, A., Olshen, A. B., Gerald, W. L., and Massague, J. (2005). Genes that mediate breast cancer metastasis to lung. Nature *436*, 518-524.

Miralles, F., Posern, G., Zaromytidou, A. I., and Treisman, R. (2003). Actin dynamics control SRF activity by regulation of its coactivator MAL. Cell *113*, 329-342.

Morgan, M. R., Hamidi, H., Bass, M. D., Warwood, S., Ballestrem, C., and Humphries, M. J. (2013). Syndecan-4 phosphorylation is a control point for integrin recycling. Dev Cell *24*, 472-485.

Mori, M., Muramatsu, Y., Yamada, K., Shrestha, P., and Takai, Y. (1996). Intracellular localization of tenascin in squamous cell carcinoma of oral cavity: an immunohistochemical study. Anticancer Res *16*, 3075-3079.

Mori, M., Yamada, T., Doi, T., Ohmura, H., Takai, Y., and Shrestha, P. (1995). Expression of tenascin in odontogenic tumours. Eur J Cancer B Oral Oncol *31B*, 275-279.

Moritz, S., Lehmann, S., Faissner, A., and von Holst, A. (2008). An induction gene trap screen in neural stem cells reveals an instructive function of the niche and identifies the splicing regulator sam68 as a tenascin-C-regulated target gene. Stem Cells *26*, 2321-2331.

Murphy-Ullrich, J. E., Lightner, V. A., Aukhil, I., Yan, Y. Z., Erickson, H. P., and Hook, M. (1991). Focal adhesion integrity is downregulated by the alternatively spliced domain of human tenascin. J Cell Biol *115*, 1127-1136.

Mustafa, D. A., Dekker, L. J., Stingl, C., Kremer, A., Stoop, M., Sillevis Smitt, P. A., Kros, J. M., and Luider, T. M. (2012). A proteome comparison between physiological angiogenesis and angiogenesis in glioblastoma. Mol Cell Proteomics *11*, M111 008466.

Nagaharu, K., Zhang, X., Yoshida, T., Katoh, D., Hanamura, N., Kozuka, Y., Ogawa, T., Shiraishi, T., and Imanaka-Yoshida, K. (2011). Tenascin C induces epithelial-mesenchymal transition-like change accompanied by SRC activation and focal adhesion kinase phosphorylation in human breast cancer cells. Am J Pathol *178*, 754-763.

Nagata, M., Fujita, H., Ida, H., Hoshina, H., Inoue, T., Seki, Y., Ohnishi, M., Ohyama, T., Shingaki, S., Kaji, M., *et al.* (2003). Identification of potential biomarkers of lymph node metastasis in oral squamous cell carcinoma by cDNA microarray analysis. Int J Cancer *106*, 683-689.

Nakahara, H., Gabazza, E. C., Fujimoto, H., Nishii, Y., D'Alessandro-Gabazza, C. N., Bruno, N. E., Takagi, T., Hayashi, T., Maruyama, J., Maruyama, K., *et al.* (2006). Deficiency of tenascin C attenuates allergen-induced bronchial asthma in the mouse. Eur J Immunol *36*, 3334-3345.

Natali, P. G., Nicotra, M. R., Bartolazzi, A., Mottolese, M., Coscia, N., Bigotti, A., and Zardi, L. (1990). Expression and production of tenascin in benign and malignant lesions of melanocyte lineage. Int J Cancer *46*, 586-590.

O'Brien, J., Hansen, K., Barkan, D., Green, J., Schedin, P., O'Brien, J., Hansen, K., Barkan, D., Green, J., and Schedin, P. (2011). Non-steroidal anti-inflammatory drugs target the pro-tumorigenic extracellular matrix of the postpartum mammary gland. Int J Dev Biol *55*, 745-755.

O'Connell, J. T., Sugimoto, H., Cooke, V. G., MacDonald, B. A., Mehta, A. I., LeBleu, V. S., Dewar, R., Rocha, R. M., Brentani, R. R., Resnick, M. B., *et al.* (2011). VEGF-A and Tenascin-C produced by S100A4+ stromal cells are important for metastatic colonization. Proc Natl Acad Sci U S A *108*, 16002-16007.

Ohno, Y., Izumi, M., Yoshioka, K., Ohori, M., Yonou, H., and Tachibana, M. (2008). Prognostic significance of tenascin-C expression in clear cell renal cell carcinoma. Oncol Rep *20*, 511-516.

Ohta, M., Sakai, T., Saga, Y., Aizawa, S., and Saito, M. (1998). Suppression of hematopoietic activity in tenascin-C-deficient mice. Blood *91*, 4074-4083.

Okano, H., Kawahara, H., Toriya, M., Nakao, K., Shibata, S., and Imai, T. (2005). Function of RNA-binding protein Musashi-1 in stem cells. Exp Cell Res *306*, 349-356.

Olson, E. N., and Nordheim, A. (2010). Linking actin dynamics and gene transcription to drive cellular motile functions. Nat Rev Mol Cell Biol 11, 353-365.

Olsson, A. K., and Hellman, L. (2011). A novel vaccine that targets tumor vessels as an efficient tool in tumor therapy. Patent number: WO/2011/075035.

Orend, G. (2005). Potential oncogenic action of tenascin-C in tumorigenesis. Int J Biochem Cell Biol 37, 1066-1083.

Orend, G., and Chiquet-Ehrismann, R. (2006). Tenascin-C induced signaling in cancer. Cancer Lett 244, 143-163.

Orend, G., Huang, W., Olayioye, M. A., Hynes, N. E., and Chiquet-Ehrismann, R. (2003). Tenascin-C blocks cell-cycle progression of anchorage-dependent fibroblasts on fibronectin through inhibition of syndecan-4. Oncogene 22, 3917-3926.

Oskarsson, T., Acharyya, S., Zhang, X. H., Vanharanta, S., Tavazoie, S. F., Morris, P. G., Downey, R. J., Manova-Todorova, K., Brogi, E., and Massague, J. (2011). Breast cancer cells produce tenascin C as a metastatic niche component to colonize the lungs. Nat Med 17, 867-874.

Oskarsson, T., and Massague, J. (2012). Extracellular matrix players in metastatic niches. EMBO J 31, 254-256.

Oz, B., Karayel, F. A., Gazio, N. L., Ozlen, F., and Balci, K. (2000). The distribution of extracellular matrix proteins and CD44S expression in human astrocytomas. Pathol Oncol Res 6, 118-124.

Paez-Ribes, M., Allen, E., Hudock, J., Takeda, T., Okuyama, H., Vinals, F., Inoue, M., Bergers, G., Hanahan, D., and Casanovas, O. (2009). Antiangiogenic therapy elicits malignant progression of tumors to increased local invasion and distant metastasis. Cancer Cell 15, 220-231.

Paganelli, G., Bartolomei, M., Ferrari, M., Cremonesi, M., Broggi, G., Maira, G., Sturiale, C., Grana, C., Prisco, G., Gatti, M., et al. (2001). Pre-targeted locoregional radioimmunotherapy with 90Y-biotin in glioma patients: phase I study and preliminary therapeutic results. Cancer Biother Radiopharm 16, 227-235.

Paget, S. (1889). The distribution of secondary growths in cancer of the breast. The Lancet *133*, 571-573.

Paget, S. (1989). The distribution of secondary growths in cancer of the breast. 1889. Cancer Metastasis Rev *8*, 98-101.

Parekh, K., Ramachandran, S., Cooper, J., Bigner, D., Patterson, A., and Mohanakumar, T. (2005). Tenascin-C, over expressed in lung cancer down regulates effector functions of tumor infiltrating lymphocytes. Lung Cancer *47*, 17-29.

Pas, J., Wyszko, E., Rolle, K., Rychlewski, L., Nowak, S., Zukiel, R., and Barciszewski, J. (2006). Analysis of structure and function of tenascin-C. Int J Biochem Cell Biol *38*, 1594-1602.

Patel, L., Sun, W., Glasson, S. S., Morris, E. A., Flannery, C. R., and Chockalingam, P. S. (2011). Tenascin-C induces inflammatory mediators and matrix degradation in osteoarthritic cartilage. BMC Musculoskelet Disord *12*, 164.

Pauli, C., Stieber, P., Schmitt, U. M., Andratschke, M., Hoffmann, K., and Wollenberg, B. (2002). The significance of Tenascin-C serum level as tumor marker in squamous cell carcinoma of the head and neck. Anticancer Res *22*, 3093-3097.

Pazzaglia, L., Conti, A., Chiechi, A., Novello, C., Magagnoli, G., Astolfi, A., Pession, A., Krenacs, T., Alberghini, M., Picci, P., and Benassi, M. S. (2010). Differential gene expression in classic giant cell tumours of bone: Tenascin C as biological risk factor for local relapses and metastases. Histopathology *57*, 59-72.

Pedretti, M., Soltermann, A., Arni, S., Weder, W., Neri, D., and Hillinger, S. (2009). Comparative immunohistochemistry of L19 and F16 in non-small cell lung cancer and mesothelioma: two human antibodies investigated in clinical trials in patients with cancer. Lung Cancer *64*, 28-33.

Pedretti, M., Verpelli, C., Marlind, J., Bertani, G., Sala, C., Neri, D., and Bello, L. (2010). Combination of temozolomide with immunocytokine F16-IL2 for the treatment of glioblastoma. Br J Cancer *103*, 827-836.

Persson, O., Krogh, M., Saal, L. H., Englund, E., Liu, J., Parsons, R., Mandahl, N., Borg, A., Widegren, B., and Salford, L. G. (2007). Microarray analysis of gliomas reveals chromosomal position-associated gene expression patterns and identifies potential immunotherapy targets. J Neurooncol *85*, 11-24.

Petronzelli, F., Pelliccia, A., Anastasi, A. M., D'Alessio, V., Albertoni, C., Rosi, A., Leoni, B., De Angelis, C., Paganelli, G., Palombo, G., *et al.* (2005). Improved tumor targeting by combined use of two antitenascin antibodies. Clin Cancer Res *11*, 7137s-7145s.

Pezzolo, A., Parodi, F., Marimpietri, D., Raffaghello, L., Cocco, C., Pistorio, A., Mosconi, M., Gambini, C., Cilli, M., Deaglio, S., *et al.* (2011). Oct-4+/Tenascin C+ neuroblastoma cells serve as progenitors of tumor-derived endothelial cells. Cell Res *21*, 1470-1486.

Piccinini, A. M., and Midwood, K. (2012). Endogenous Control of Immunity against Infection: Tenascin-C Regulates TLR4-Mediated Inflammation via MicroRNA-155. Cell reports *In press*.

Pilch, H., Schaffer, U., Schlenger, K., Lautz, A., Tanner, B., Hockel, M., and Knapstein, P. G. (1999). Expression of tenascin in human cervical cancer--association of tenascin expression with clinicopathological parameters. Gynecol Oncol *73*, 415-421.

Pollanen, R., Soini, Y., Vuopala, S., Laara, E., and Lehto, V. P. (1996). Tenascin in human papillomavirus associated lesions of the uterine cervix. J Clin Pathol *49*, 521-523.

Prieto, A. L., Edelman, G. M., and Crossin, K. L. (1993). Multiple integrins mediate cell attachment to cytotactin/tenascin. Proc Natl Acad Sci U S A *90*, 10154-10158.

Probstmeier, R., and Pesheva, P. (1999). Tenascin-C inhibits beta1 integrin-dependent cell adhesion and neurite outgrowth on fibronectin by a disialoganglioside-mediated signaling mechanism. Glycobiology *9*, 101-114.

Procopio, A., Strizzi, L., Giuffrida, A., Scarpa, S., Giuliano, M., Iezzi, T., Mutti, L., and Modesti, A. (1998). Human malignant mesothelioma of the pleura: new perspectives for diagnosis and therapy. Monaldi Arch Chest Dis *53*, 241-243.

Psaila, B., and Lyden, D. (2009). The metastatic niche: adapting the foreign soil. Nat Rev Cancer *9*, 285-293.

Qian, X., Shen, Q., Goderie, S. K., He, W., Capela, A., Davis, A. A., and Temple, S. (2000). Timing of CNS cell generation: a programmed sequence of neuron and glial cell production from isolated murine cortical stem cells. Neuron *28*, 69-80.

Ramaswamy, S., Ross, K. N., Lander, E. S., and Golub, T. R. (2003). A molecular signature of metastasis in primary solid tumors. Nat Genet *33*, 49-54.

Rauch, U., Feng, K., and Zhou, X. H. (2001). Neurocan: a brain chondroitin sulfate proteoglycan. Cell Mol Life Sci *58*, 1842-1856.

Reardon, D. A., Akabani, G., Coleman, R. E., Friedman, A. H., Friedman, H. S., Herndon, J. E., 2nd, McLendon, R. E., Pegram, C. N., Provenzale, J. M., Quinn, J. A., *et al.* (2006). Salvage radioimmunotherapy with murine iodine-131-labeled antitenascin monoclonal antibody 81C6 for patients with recurrent primary and metastatic malignant brain tumors: phase II study results. J Clin Oncol *24*, 115-122.

Reardon, D. A., Zalutsky, M. R., Akabani, G., Coleman, R. E., Friedman, A. H., Herndon, J. E., 2nd, McLendon, R. E., Pegram, C. N., Quinn, J. A., Rich, J. N., *et al.* (2008). A pilot study: 131I-antitenascin monoclonal antibody 81c6 to deliver a 44-Gy resection cavity boost. Neuro Oncol *10*, 182-189.

Redick, S. D., and Schwarzbauer, J. E. (1995). Rapid intracellular assembly of tenascin hexabrachions suggests a novel cotranslational process. J Cell Sci *108 ( Pt 4)*, 1761-1769.

Regezi, J. A., Ramos, D. M., Pytela, R., Dekker, N. P., and Jordan, R. C. (2002). Tenascin and beta 6 integrin are overexpressed in floor of mouth in situ carcinomas and invasive squamous cell carcinomas. Oral Oncol *38*, 332-336.

Reilly, R. M. (2010). Monoclonal Antibody and Peptide-Targeted Radiotherapy of Cancer. Wiley VCH; Book chapter 54.

Reinertsen, T., Halgunset, J., Viset, T., Flatberg, A., Haugsmoen, L. L., and Skogseth, H. (2012). Gene expressional changes in prostate fibroblasts from cancerous tissue. Apmis *120*, 558-571.

Ren, S., Johnson, B. G., Kida, Y., Ip, C., Davidson, K. C., Lin, S. L., Kobayashi, A., Lang, R. A., Hadjantonakis, A. K., Moon, R. T., and Duffield, J. S. (2013). LRP-6 is a coreceptor for multiple fibrogenic signaling pathways in pericytes and myofibroblasts that are inhibited by DKK-1. Proc Natl Acad Sci U S A *110*, 1440-1445.

Renkonen, S., Heikkila, P., Haglund, C., Makitie, A. A., and Hagstrom, J. (2012). Tenascin-C, GLUT-1, and syndecan-2 expression in juvenile nasopharyngeal angiofibroma: Correlations to vessel density and tumor stage. Head Neck.

Reya, T., Morrison, S. J., Clarke, M. F., and Weissman, I. L. (2001). Stem cells, cancer, and cancer stem cells. Nature 414, 105-111.

Ricci-Vitiani, L., Pallini, R., Biffoni, M., Todaro, M., Invernici, G., Cenci, T., Maira, G., Parati, E. A., Stassi, G., Larocca, L. M., and De Maria, R. (2010). Tumour vascularization via endothelial differentiation of glioblastoma stem-like cells. Nature 468, 824-828.

Richter, P., Tost, M., Franz, M., Altendorf-Hofmann, A., Junker, K., Borsi, L., Neri, D., Kosmehl, H., Wunderlich, H., and Berndt, A. (2009). B and C domain containing tenascin-C: urinary markers for invasiveness of urothelial carcinoma of the urinary bladder? J Cancer Res Clin Oncol 135, 1351-1358.

Riedl, S., Bodenmuller, H., Hinz, U., Holle, R., Moller, P., Schlag, P., Herfarth, C., and Faissner, A. (1995). Significance of tenascin serum level as tumor marker in primary colorectal carcinoma. Int J Cancer 64, 65-69.

Riedl, S., Tandara, A., Reinshagen, M., Hinz, U., Faissner, A., Bodenmuller, H., Buhr, H. J., Herfarth, C., and Moller, P. (2001). Serum tenascin-C is an indicator of inflammatory bowel disease activity. Int J Colorectal Dis 16, 285-291.

Riedl, S. E., Faissner, A., Schlag, P., Von Herbay, A., Koretz, K., and Moller, P. (1992). Altered content and distribution of tenascin in colitis, colon adenoma, and colorectal carcinoma. Gastroenterology 103, 400-406.

Riva, P., Arista, A., Tison, V., Sturiale, C., Franceschi, G., Spinelli, A., Riva, N., Casi, M., Moscatelli, G., and Frattarelli, M. (1994). Intralesional radioimmunotherapy of malignant gliomas. An effective treatment in recurrent tumors. Cancer 73, 1076-1082.

Rolle, K., Nowak, S., Wyszko, E., Nowak, M., Zukiel, R., Piestrzeniewicz, R., Gawronska, I., Barciszewska, M. Z., and Barciszewski, J. (2010). Promising human brain tumors therapy with interference RNA intervention (iRNAi). Cancer Biol Ther 9, 396-406.

Ruggiero, S., Cosgarea, R., Potempa, J., Potempa, B., Eick, S., and Chiquet, M. (2013). Cleavage of extracellular matrix in periodontitis: gingipains differentially affect cell adhesion activities of fibronectin and tenascin-C. Biochim Biophys Acta 1832, 517-526.

Ruhmann, M., Piccinini, A. M., Kong, P. L., and Midwood, K. S. (2012). Endogenous activation of adaptive immunity: tenascin-C drives interleukin-17 synthesis in murine arthritic joint disease. Arthritis Rheum 64, 2179-2190.

Ruiz, C., Huang, W., Hegi, M. E., Lange, K., Hamou, M. F., Fluri, E., Oakeley, E. J., Chiquet-Ehrismann, R., and Orend, G. (2004). Growth promoting signaling by tenascin-C [corrected]. Cancer Res 64, 7377-7385.

Saga, Y., Yagi, T., Ikawa, Y., Sakakura, T., and Aizawa, S. (1992). Mice develop normally without tenascin. Genes Dev 6, 1821-1831.

Saito, Y., Imazeki, H., Miura, S., Yoshimura, T., Okutsu, H., Harada, Y., Ohwaki, T., Nagao, O., Kamiya, S., Hayashi, R., et al. (2007). A peptide derived from tenascin-C induces beta1 integrin activation through syndecan-4. J Biol Chem 282, 34929-34937.

Sakai, T., Kawakatsu, H., Hirota, N., Yokoyama, T., Sakakura, T., and Saito, M. (1993). Specific expression of tenascin in human colonic neoplasms. Br J Cancer 67, 1058-1064.

Salmenkivi, K., Haglund, C., Arola, J., and Heikkila, P. (2001). Increased expression of tenascin in pheochromocytomas correlates with malignancy. Am J Surg Pathol 25, 1419-1423.

Sampson, J. H., Akabani, G., Friedman, A. H., Bigner, D., Kunwar, S., Berger, M. S., and Bankiewicz, K. S. (2006). Comparison of intratumoral bolus injection and convection-enhanced delivery of radiolabeled antitenascin monoclonal antibodies. Neurosurg Focus 20, E14.

Sarkar, S., Nuttall, R. K., Liu, S., Edwards, D. R., and Yong, V. W. (2006). Tenascin-C stimulates glioma cell invasion through matrix metalloproteinase-12. Cancer Res 66, 11771-11780.

Sarkar, S., and Yong, V. W. (2010). Reduction of protein kinase C delta attenuates tenascin-C stimulated glioma invasion in three-dimensional matrix. Carcinogenesis 31, 311-317.

Saupe, F., Schwenzer, A., Jia, Y., Gasser, I., Spenle, C., Langlois, B., Kammerer, M., Lefebvre, O., Hlushchuk, R., Rupp, T., *et al.* (2013). Tenascin-C downregulates wnt inhibitor dickkopf-1, promoting tumorigenesis in a neuroendocrine tumor model. Cell Rep 5, 482-492.

Saxon, B. R., Byard, R. W., and Han, P. (1997). Cellular expression of adhesion factors in childhood rhabdomyosarcoma. Pediatr Pathol Lab Med 17, 259-266.

Schaff, M., Receveur, N., Bourdon, C., Wurtz, V., Denis, C. V., Orend, G., Gachet, C., Lanza, F., and Mangin, P. H. (2010). Novel function of tenascin-C, a matrix protein relevant to atherosclerosis, in platelet recruitment and activation under flow. Arterioscler Thromb Vasc Biol 31, 117-124.

Schenk, S., Chiquet-Ehrismann, R., and Battegay, E. J. (1999). The fibrinogen globe of tenascin-C promotes basic fibroblast growth factor-induced endothelial cell elongation. Mol Biol Cell 10, 2933-2943.

Schenk, S., Muser, J., Vollmer, G., and Chiquet-Ehrismann, R. (1995). Tenascin-C in serum: a questionable tumor marker. Int J Cancer 61, 443-449.

Schliemann, C., Wiedmer, A., Pedretti, M., Szczepanowski, M., Klapper, W., and Neri, D. (2009). Three clinical-stage tumor targeting antibodies reveal differential expression of oncofetal fibronectin and tenascin-C isoforms in human lymphoma. Leuk Res 33, 1718-1722.

Schmidt, K. S., Borkowski, S., Kurreck, J., Stephens, A. W., Bald, R., Hecht, M., Friebe, M., Dinkelborg, L., and Erdmann, V. A. (2004). Application of locked nucleic acids to improve aptamer in vivo stability and targeting function. Nucleic Acids Res 32, 5757-5765.

Schnapp, L. M., Hatch, N., Ramos, D. M., Klimanskaya, I. V., Sheppard, D., and Pytela, R. (1995). The human integrin alpha 8 beta 1 functions as a receptor for tenascin, fibronectin, and vitronectin. J Biol Chem 270, 23196-23202.

Schneller, M., Vuori, K., and Ruoslahti, E. (1997). Alphavbeta3 integrin associates with activated insulin and PDGFbeta receptors and potentiates the biological activity of PDGF. Embo J 16, 5600-5607.

Schumacher, S., Jung, M., Norenberg, U., Dorner, A., Chiquet-Ehrismann, R., Stuermer, C. A., and Rathjen, F. G. (2001). CALEB binds via its acidic stretch to the fibrinogen-like domain of tenascin-C or tenascin-R and its expression is dynamically regulated after optic nerve lesion. J Biol Chem *276*, 7337-7345.

Schwager, K., Villa, A., Rosli, C., Neri, D., Rosli-Khabas, M., and Moser, G. (2011). A comparative immunofluorescence analysis of three clinical-stage antibodies in head and neck cancer. Head Neck Oncol *3*, 25.

Seiffert, M., Beck, S. C., Schermutzki, F., Muller, C. A., Erickson, H. P., and Klein, G. (1998). Mitogenic and adhesive effects of tenascin-C on human hematopoietic cells are mediated by various functional domains. Matrix Biol *17*, 47-63.

Seo, E., Basu-Roy, U., Gunaratne, P. H., Coarfa, C., Lim, D. S., Basilico, C., and Mansukhani, A. (2013). SOX2 Regulates YAP1 to Maintain Stemness and Determine Cell Fate in the Osteo-Adipo Lineage. Cell Rep *3*, 2075-2087.

Shah, C., Miller, T. W., Wyatt, S. K., McKinley, E. T., Olivares, M. G., Sanchez, V., Nolting, D. D., Buck, J. R., Zhao, P., Ansari, M. S., et al. (2009). Imaging biomarkers predict response to anti-HER2 (ErbB2) therapy in preclinical models of breast cancer. Clin Cancer Res *15*, 4712-4721.

Shang, B., Cao, Z., and Zhou, Q. (2012). Progress in tumor vascular normalization for anticancer therapy: challenges and perspectives. Front Med *6*, 67-78.

Shintani, S., Alcalde, R. E., Matsumura, T., and Terakado, N. (1997). Extracellular matrices expression in invasion area of adenoid cystic carcinoma of salivary glands. Cancer Lett *116*, 9-14.

Shoji, T., Kamiya, T., Tsubura, A., Hamada, Y., Hatano, T., Hioki, K., and Morii, S. (1993). Tenascin staining positivity and the survival of patients with invasive breast carcinoma. J Surg Res *55*, 295-297.

Shrestha, P., Sakamoto, F., Takagi, H., Yamada, T., and Mori, M. (1994). Enhanced tenascin immunoreactivity in leukoplakia and squamous cell carcinoma of the oral cavity: an immunohistochemical study. Eur J Cancer B Oral Oncol *30B*, 132-137.

Silacci, M., Brack, S. S., Spath, N., Buck, A., Hillinger, S., Arni, S., Weder, W., Zardi, L., and Neri, D. (2006). Human monoclonal antibodies to domain C of tenascin-C selectively target solid tumors in vivo. Protein Eng Des Sel *19*, 471-478.

Sis, B., Sagol, O., Kupelioglu, A., Sokmen, S., Terzi, C., Fuzun, M., Ozer, E., and Bishop, P. (2004). Prognostic significance of matrix metalloproteinase-2, cathepsin D, and tenascin-C expression in colorectal carcinoma. Pathol Res Pract *200*, 379-387.

Sobocinski, G. P., Toy, K., Bobrowski, W. F., Shaw, S., Anderson, A. O., and Kaldjian, E. P. (2010). Ultrastructural localization of extracellular matrix proteins of the lymph node cortex: evidence supporting the reticular network as a pathway for lymphocyte migration. BMC Immunol *11*, 42.

Soini, Y., Paakko, P., Nuorva, K., Kamel, D., Linnala, A., Virtanen, I., and Lehto, V. P. (1993). Tenascin immunoreactivity in lung tumors. Am J Clin Pathol *100*, 145-150.

Spring, J., Beck, K., and Chiquet-Ehrismann, R. (1989). Two contrary functions of tenascin: dissection of the active sites by recombinant tenascin fragments. Cell *59*, 325-334.

Srinivasan, J., Schachner, M., and Catterall, W. A. (1998). Interaction of voltage-gated sodium channels with the extracellular matrix molecules tenascin-C and tenascin-R. Proc Natl Acad Sci U S A *95*, 15753-15757.

Sriramarao, P., and Bourdon, M. A. (1993). A novel tenascin type III repeat is part of a complex of tenascin mRNA alternative splices. Nucleic Acids Res *21*, 163-168.

Sriramarao, P., Mendler, M., and Bourdon, M. A. (1993). Endothelial cell attachment and spreading on human tenascin is mediated by alpha 2 beta 1 and alpha v beta 3 integrins. J Cell Sci *105 ( Pt 4)*, 1001-1012.

Sugawara, I., Hirakoshi, J., Masunaga, A., Itoyama, S., and Sakakura, T. (1991). Reduced tenascin expression in colonic carcinoma with lymphogenous metastasis. Invasion Metastasis *11*, 325-331.

Sumioka, T., Fujita, N., Kitano, A., Okada, Y., and Saika, S. (2011). Impaired angiogenic response in the cornea of mice lacking tenascin C. Invest Ophthalmol Vis Sci *52*, 2462-2467.

Suwiwat, S., Ricciardelli, C., Tammi, R., Tammi, M., Auvinen, P., Kosma, V. M., LeBaron, R. G., Raymond, W. A., Tilley, W. D., and Horsfall,

D. J. (2004). Expression of extracellular matrix components versican, chondroitin sulfate, tenascin, and hyaluronan, and their association with disease outcome in node-negative breast cancer. Clin Cancer Res *10*, 2491-2498.

Swindle, C. S., Tran, K. T., Johnson, T. D., Banerjee, P., Mayes, A. M., Griffith, L., and Wells, A. (2001). Epidermal growth factor (EGF)-like repeats of human tenascin-C as ligands for EGF receptor. J Cell Biol *154*, 459-468.

Takeda, A., Otani, Y., Hirooka, E., Okada, K., Torii, T., Shinozuka, N., and Koyama, I. (2007). Plasma large Tenascin-C spliced variant as a possible biomarker for the prediction of hepatic recurrence in colorectal cancer. Surgery *141*, 124-125.

Talts, J. F., Wirl, G., Dictor, M., Muller, W. J., and Fassler, R. (1999). Tenascin-C modulates tumor stroma and monocyte/macrophage recruitment but not tumor growth or metastasis in a mouse strain with spontaneous mammary cancer. J Cell Sci *112 ( Pt 12)*, 1855-1864.

Tanaka, F., Otake, Y., Yanagihara, K., Kawano, Y., Miyahara, R., Li, M., Yamada, T., Hanaoka, N., Inui, K., and Wada, H. (2001). Evaluation of angiogenesis in non-small cell lung cancer: comparison between anti-CD34 antibody and anti-CD105 antibody. Clin Cancer Res *7*, 3410-3415.

Tanaka, K., Hiraiwa, N., Hashimoto, H., Yamazaki, Y., and Kusakabe, M. (2004). Tenascin-C regulates angiogenesis in tumor through the regulation of vascular endothelial growth factor expression. Int J Cancer *108*, 31-40.

Tanaka, M., Yamazaki, T., Araki, N., Yoshikawa, H., Yoshida, T., Sakakura, T., and Uchida, A. (2000). Clinical significance of tenascin-C expression in osteosarcoma: tenascin-C promotes distant metastases of osteosarcoma. Int J Mol Med *5*, 505-510.

Tanaka, R., Owaki, T., Kamiya, S., Matsunaga, T., Shimoda, K., Kodama, H., Hayashi, R., Abe, T., Harada, Y. P., Shimonaka, M., *et al.* (2009). VLA-5-mediated adhesion to fibronectin accelerates hemin-stimulated erythroid differentiation of K562 cells through induction of VLA-4 expression. J Biol Chem *284*, 19817-19825.

Tanaka, S., Sumioka, T., Fujita, N., Kitano, A., Okada, Y., Yamanaka, O., Flanders, K. C., Miyajima, M., and Saika, S. (2010). Suppression of injury-induced epithelial-mesenchymal transition in a mouse lens epithelium lacking tenascin-C. Mol Vis *16*, 1194-1205.

Taraseviciute, A., Vincent, B. T., Schedin, P., and Jones, P. L. (2010). Quantitative analysis of three-dimensional human mammary epithelial tissue architecture reveals a role for tenascin-C in regulating c-met function. Am J Pathol *176*, 827-838.

Tavazoie, S. F., Alarcon, C., Oskarsson, T., Padua, D., Wang, Q., Bos, P. D., Gerald, W. L., and Massague, J. (2008). Endogenous human microRNAs that suppress breast cancer metastasis. Nature *451*, 147-152.

Taylor, H. C., Lightner, V. A., Beyer, W. F., Jr., McCaslin, D., Briscoe, G., and Erickson, H. P. (1989). Biochemical and structural studies of tenascin/hexabrachion proteins. J Cell Biochem *41*, 71-90.

Tiitta, O., Happonen, R. P., Virtanen, I., and Luomanen, M. (1994a). Distribution of tenascin in oral premalignant lesions and squamous cell carcinoma. J Oral Pathol Med *23*, 446-450.

Tiitta, O., Sipponen, P., Gould, V., and Virtanen, I. (1994b). Tenascin expression in inflammatory, dysplastic and neoplastic lesions of the human stomach. Virchows Arch *425*, 369-374.

Tiitta, O., Wahlstrom, T., Virtanen, I., and Gould, V. E. (1993). Tenascin in inflammatory conditions and neoplasms of the urinary bladder. Virchows Arch B Cell Pathol Incl Mol Pathol *63*, 283-287.

To, W. S., and Midwood, K. S. (2010). Cryptic domains of tenascin-C differentially control fibronectin fibrillogenesis. Matrix Biol *29*, 573-585.

To, W. S., and Midwood, K. S. (2011). Identification of novel and distinct binding sites within tenascin-C for soluble and fibrillar fibronectin. J Biol Chem *286*, 14881-14891.

Tokes, A. M., Hortovanyi, E., Csordas, G., Kulka, J., Mozes, G., Hatalyak, A., and Kadar, A. (1999). Immunohistochemical localisation of tenascin in invasive ductal carcinoma of the breast. Anticancer Res *19*, 175-179.

Tremblay, G. A., and Richard, S. (2006). mRNAs associated with the Sam68 RNA binding protein. RNA Biol *3*, 90-93.

Tsunoda, T., Inada, H., Kalembeyi, I., Imanaka-Yoshida, K., Sakakibara, M., Okada, R., Katsuta, K., Sakakura, T., Majima, Y., and Yoshida, T. (2003). Involvement of large tenascin-C splice variants in breast cancer progression. Am J Pathol *162*, 1857-1867.

Tucker, R. P., and Chiquet-Ehrismann, R. (2009). The regulation of tenascin expression by tissue microenvironments. Biochim Biophys Acta *1793*, 888-892.

Tuerk, C., MacDougal, S., and Gold, L. (1992). RNA pseudoknots that inhibit human immunodeficiency virus type 1 reverse transcriptase. Proc Natl Acad Sci U S A *89*, 6988-6992.

Tumova, S., Woods, A., and Couchman, J. R. (2000). Heparan sulfate chains from glypican and syndecans bind the Hep II domain of fibronectin similarly despite minor structural differences. J Biol Chem *275*, 9410-9417.

Tuominen, H., and Kallioinen, M. (1994). Increased tenascin expression in melanocytic tumors. J Cutan Pathol *21*, 424-429.

Udalova, I. A., Ruhmann, M., Thomson, S. J., and Midwood, K. S. (2011). Expression and immune function of tenascin-C. Crit Rev Immunol *31*, 115-145.

Uhlman, D. L., and Niehans, G. A. (1999). Immunohistochemical study of chondroitin-6-sulphate and tenascin in the larynx: a loss of chondroitin-6-sulphate expression accompanies squamous cell carcinoma invasion. J Pathol *189*, 470-474.

Vaidya, P., Yosida, T., Sakakura, T., Yatani, R., Noguchi, T., and Kawarada, Y. (1996). Combined analysis of expression of c-erbB-2, Ki-67 antigen, and tenascin provides a better prognostic indicator of carcinoma of the papilla of Vater. Pancreas *12*, 196-201.

Van Obberghen-Schilling, E., Tucker, R. P., Saupe, F., Gasser, I., Cseh, B., and Orend, G. (2011a). Fibronectin and tenascin-C: accomplices in vascular morphogenesis during development and tumor growth. The International journal of developmental biology *55*, 511-525.

Van Obberghen-Schilling, E., Tucker, R. P., Saupe, F., Gasser, I., Cseh, B., and Orend, G. (2011b). Fibronectin and tenascin-C: accomplices in vascular morphogenesis during development and tumor growth. Int J Dev Biol *55*, 511-525.

Varga, I., Hutoczki, G., Szemcsak, C. D., Zahuczky, G., Toth, J., Adamecz, Z., Kenyeres, A., Bognar, L., Hanzely, Z., and Klekner, A. (2012). Brevican, neurocan, tenascin-C and versican are mainly responsible for the invasiveness of low-grade astrocytoma. Pathol Oncol Res 18, 413-420.

Vaughan, L., Weber, P., D'Alessandri, L., Zisch, A. H., and Winterhalter, K. H. (1994). Tenascin-contactin/F11 interactions: a clue for a developmental role? Perspect Dev Neurobiol 2, 43-52.

Veillet, A. L., Haag, J. D., Remfert, J. L., Meilahn, A. L., Samuelson, D. J., and Gould, M. N. (2011). Mcs5c: a mammary carcinoma susceptibility locus located in a gene desert that associates with tenascin C expression. Cancer Prev Res (Phila) 4, 97-106.

Verstraeten, A. A., Mackie, E. J., Hageman, P. C., Hilgers, J., Schol, D. J., De Jongh, G. J., and Schalkwijk, J. (1992). Tenascin expression in basal cell carcinoma. Br J Dermatol 127, 571-574.

Viale, G. L., Castellani, P., Dorcaratto, A., Pau, A., Sehrbundt, E., Siri, A., Biro, A., and Zardi, L. (2002). Occurrence of a glioblastoma-associated tenascin-C isoform in cerebral cavernomas and neighboring vessels. Neurosurgery 50, 838-842; discussion 842.

Vollmer, G., Siegal, G. P., Chiquet-Ehrismann, R., Lightner, V. A., Arnholdt, H., and Knuppen, R. (1990). Tenascin expression in the human endometrium and in endometrial adenocarcinomas. Lab Invest 62, 725-730.

Vollmer, T., Hinse, D., Kleesiek, K., and Dreier, J. (2010). Interactions between endocarditis-derived Streptococcus gallolyticus subsp. gallolyticus isolates and human endothelial cells. BMC Microbiol 10, 78.

von Holst, A., Egbers, U., Prochiantz, A., and Faissner, A. (2007). Neural stem/progenitor cells express 20 tenascin C isoforms that are differentially regulated by Pax6. J Biol Chem 282, 9172-9181.

Vredenburgh, J. J., Desjardins, A., Herndon, J. E., 2nd, Marcello, J., Reardon, D. A., Quinn, J. A., Rich, J. N., Sathornsumetee, S., Gururangan, S., Sampson, J., et al. (2007). Bevacizumab plus irinotecan in recurrent glioblastoma multiforme. J Clin Oncol 25, 4722-4729.

Wang, L., Wang, W., Shah, P. K., Song, L., Yang, M., and Sharifi, B. G. (2012). Deletion of tenascin-C gene exacerbates atherosclerosis and induces intraplaque hemorrhage in Apo-E-deficient mice. Cardiovasc Pathol 21, 398-413.

Wang, R., Chadalavada, K., Wilshire, J., Kowalik, U., Hovinga, K. E., Geber, A., Fligelman, B., Leversha, M., Brennan, C., and Tabar, V. (2010a). Glioblastoma stem-like cells give rise to tumour endothelium. Nature 468, 829-833.

Wang, Z., Han, B., Zhang, Z., Pan, J., and Xia, H. (2010b). Expression of angiopoietin-like 4 and tenascin C but not cathepsin C mRNA predicts prognosis of oral tongue squamous cell carcinoma. Biomarkers 15, 39-46.

Weber, P., Zimmermann, D. R., Winterhalter, K. H., and Vaughan, L. (1995). Tenascin-C binds heparin by its fibronectin type III domain five. J Biol Chem 270, 4619-4623.

Weissleder, R. (2006). Molecular imaging in cancer. Science 312, 1168-1171.

Wenk, M. B., Midwood, K. S., and Schwarzbauer, J. E. (2000). Tenascin-C suppresses Rho activation. J Cell Biol 150, 913-920.

WHO (2008). World Cancer Report 2008. International Agency for Research on Cancer, ISBN 978 92 832 0423 7.

Wijelath, E. S., Rahman, S., Namekata, M., Murray, J., Nishimura, T., Mostafavi-Pour, Z., Patel, Y., Suda, Y., Humphries, M. J., and Sobel, M. (2006). Heparin-II domain of fibronectin is a vascular endothelial growth factor-binding domain: enhancement of VEGF biological activity by a singular growth factor/matrix protein synergism. Circ Res 99, 853-860.

Wikman, H., Kettunen, E., Seppanen, J. K., Karjalainen, A., Hollmen, J., Anttila, S., and Knuutila, S. (2002). Identification of differentially expressed genes in pulmonary adenocarcinoma by using cDNA array. Oncogene 21, 5804-5813.

Wiksten, J. P., Lundin, J., Nordling, S., Lundin, M., Kokkola, A., von Boguslawski, K., and Haglund, C. (2003). Tenascin-C expression correlates with prognosis in gastric cancer. Oncology 64, 245-250.

Williams, S. A., and Schwarzbauer, J. E. (2009). A shared mechanism of adhesion modulation for tenascin-C and fibulin-1. Mol Biol Cell 20, 1141-1149.

Wilson, K. E., Langdon, S. P., Lessells, A. M., and Miller, W. R. (1996). Expression of the extracellular matrix protein tenascin in malignant and benign ovarian tumours. Br J Cancer 74, 999-1004.

Wood, C., Srivastava, P., Bukowski, R., Lacombe, L., Gorelov, A. I., Gorelov, S., Mulders, P., Zielinski, H., Hoos, A., Teofilovici, F., et al. (2008). An adjuvant autologous therapeutic vaccine (HSPPC-96; vitespen) versus observation alone for patients at high risk of recurrence after nephrectomy for renal cell carcinoma: a multicentre, open-label, randomised phase III trial. Lancet 372, 145-154.

Woods, A., and Couchman, J. R. (1994). Syndecan 4 heparan sulfate proteoglycan is a selectively enriched and widespread focal adhesion component. Mol Biol Cell 5, 183-192.

Wyszko, E., Rolle, K., Nowak, S., Zukiel, R., Nowak, M., Piestrzeniewicz, R., Gawronska, I., Barciszewska, M. Z., and Barciszewski, J. (2008). A multivariate analysis of patients with brain tumors treated with ATN-RNA. Acta Pol Pharm 65, 677-684.

Xue, Y., Li, J., Latijnhouwers, M. A., Smedts, F., Umbas, R., Aalders, T. W., Debruyne, F. M., De La Rosette, J. J., and Schalken, J. A. (1998a). Expression of periglandular tenascin-C and basement membrane laminin in normal prostate, benign prostatic hyperplasia and prostate carcinoma. Br J Urol 81, 844-851.

Xue, Y., Smedts, F., Latijnhouwers, M. A., Ruijter, E. T., Aalders, T. W., de la Rosette, J. J., Debruyne, F. M., and Schalken, J. A. (1998b). Tenascin-C expression in prostatic intraepithelial neoplasia (PIN): a marker of progression? Anticancer Res 18, 2679-2684.

Yagi, H., Yanagisawa, M., Suzuki, Y., Nakatani, Y., Ariga, T., Kato, K., and Yu, R. K. (2010). HNK-1 epitope-carrying tenascin-C spliced variant regulates the proliferation of mouse embryonic neural stem cells. J Biol Chem 285, 37293-37301.

Yokosaki, Y., Monis, H., Chen, J., and Sheppard, D. (1996). Differential effects of the integrins alpha9beta1, alphavbeta3, and alphavbeta6 on cell proliferative responses to tenascin. Roles of the beta subunit extracellular and cytoplasmic domains. J Biol Chem *271*, 24144-24150.

Yokoyama, K., Erickson, H. P., Ikeda, Y., and Takada, Y. (2000). Identification of amino acid sequences in fibrinogen gamma -chain and tenascin C C-terminal domains critical for binding to integrin alpha vbeta 3. J Biol Chem *275*, 16891-16898.

Yoshida, J., Wakabayashi, T., Okamoto, S., Kimura, S., Washizu, K., Kiyosawa, K., and Mokuno, K. (1994). Tenascin in cerebrospinal fluid is a useful biomarker for the diagnosis of brain tumour. J Neurol Neurosurg Psychiatry *57*, 1212-1215.

Yoshida, T., Matsumoto, E., Hanamura, N., Kalembeyi, I., Katsuta, K., Ishihara, A., and Sakakura, T. (1997). Co-expression of tenascin and fibronectin in epithelial and stromal cells of benign lesions and ductal carcinomas in the human breast. J Pathol *182*, 421-428.

Yoshida, T., Yoshimura, E., Numata, H., Sakakura, Y., and Sakakura, T. (1999). Involvement of tenascin-C in proliferation and migration of laryngeal carcinoma cells. Virchows Arch *435*, 496-500.

Zagzag, D., Friedlander, D. R., Dosik, J., Chikramane, S., Chan, W., Greco, M. A., Allen, J. C., Dorovini-Zis, K., and Grumet, M. (1996). Tenascin-C expression by angiogenic vessels in human astrocytomas and by human brain endothelial cells in vitro. Cancer Res *56*, 182-189.

Zagzag, D., Friedlander, D. R., Miller, D. C., Dosik, J., Cangiarella, J., Kostianovsky, M., Cohen, H., Grumet, M., and Greco, M. A. (1995). Tenascin expression in astrocytomas correlates with angiogenesis. Cancer Res *55*, 907-914.

Zagzag, D., Shiff, B., Jallo, G. I., Greco, M. A., Blanco, C., Cohen, H., Hukin, J., Allen, J. C., and Friedlander, D. R. (2002). Tenascin-C promotes microvascular cell migration and phosphorylation of focal adhesion kinase. Cancer Res *62*, 2660-2668.

Zalutsky, M. R., Reardon, D. A., Akabani, G., Coleman, R. E., Friedman, A. H., Friedman, H. S., McLendon, R. E., Wong, T. Z., and Bigner, D. D. (2008). Clinical experience with alpha-particle emitting 211At: treatment of recurrent brain tumor patients with 211At-labeled chimeric antitenascin monoclonal antibody 81C6. J Nucl Med *49*, 30-38.

Zamecnik, J., Chanova, M., Tichy, M., and Kodet, R. (2004). Distribution of the extracellular matrix glycoproteins in ependymomas--an immunohistochemical study with follow-up analysis. Neoplasma *51*, 214-222.

Zheng, H., Tsuneyama, K., Cheng, C., Takahashi, H., Cui, Z., Nomoto, K., Murai, Y., and Takano, Y. (2007). Expression of KAI1 and tenascin, and microvessel density are closely correlated with liver metastasis of gastrointestinal adenocarcinoma. J Clin Pathol *60*, 50-56.

Zirbes, T. K., Baldus, S. E., Moenig, S. P., Schmitz, K., Thiele, J., Holscher, A. H., and Dienes, H. P. (1999). Tenascin expression in gastric cancer with special emphasis on the WHO-, Lauren-, and Goseki-classifications. Int J Mol Med *4*, 39-42.

Zisch, A. H., D'Alessandri, L., Ranscht, B., Falchetto, R., Winterhalter, K. H., and Vaughan, L. (1992). Neuronal cell adhesion molecule contactin/F11 binds to tenascin via its immunoglobulin-like domains. J Cell Biol *119*, 203-213.

Zukiel, R., Nowak, S., Wyszko, E., Rolle, K., Gawronska, I., Barciszewska, M. Z., and Barciszewski, J. (2006). Suppression of human brain tumor with interference RNA specific for tenascin-C. Cancer Biol Ther *5*, 1002-1007.

Zuniga, R. M., Torcuator, R., Jain, R., Anderson, J., Doyle, T., Schultz, L., and Mikkelsen, T. (2010). Rebound tumour progression after the cessation of bevacizumab therapy in patients with recurrent high-grade glioma. J Neurooncol *99*, 237-242.

# Abbreviations

3D, three-dimensional
ANXA1, annexin 1
AML, acute myeloid leukemia
BAEC, bovine aortic endothelial cells
bFGF, basic fibroblast growth factor
BM, basement membrane
BMP, bone morphogenetic protein
BrdU, 5-bromo-2'-deoxyuridine
BREC, bovine retinal endothelial cells
BSA, bovine serum albumin
CAF, cancer associated fibroblasts
CALEB, chicken acidic leucine-rich EGF like domain containing brain protein
CMEC, cardiac microvascular endothelial cells
CNS, central nervous system
Coll, collagen
CT, computer tomography
CTGF, connective tissue growth factor
CTR, control
DAMPs, damage associated molecular patterns [DAMPs].
DKK1/2, dickkopf 1/2
DOC2, disabled homolog 2
EC, endothelial cells
ECM, extracellular matrix
EDNRA/B, endothelin receptor type A/B
EGF, epidermal growth factor
EGF-L, epidermal growth factor-like repeats
EGFR, epidermal growth factor receptor
EMT, epithelial mesenchymal transition
ET-1, endothelin-1
FAK, focal adhesion kinase

FBG, fibrinogen-like globe

FN, fibronectin

FN-EDA, fibronectin extra domain A

FN-EDB, fibronectin extra domain B

GBM, glioblastoma multiforme

GFAP, glial fibrillary acidic protein

GM7373, bovine endothelial cell line (fetal aortic endothelial cell line)

HDMEC, human microvascular endothelial cells

HEK, human embryonic kidney cells

HGF, hepatocyte growth factor

HIV, human immunodeficiency virus

HNK-1, human natural killer-1

HUVEC, human umbilical vein endothelial cells

IFN, interferon

IGF-BP, insulin-like growth factor binding proteins

IgG immunoglobulin G

IL2, interleukin-2

Kd, knock down

KO, knockout

LN, laminin

LPA, lysophosphatidic acid

LyN, lymph node

mAb, monoclonal antibody

MBP, myelin basic protein

MEF, mouse embryonic fibroblasts

miR-155, micro-RNA 155

MMP, matrix metalloprotease

MMTV, mouse mammary tumor virus

MR, magic roundabout

MRI, magnetic resonance imaging

MSl1, Musashi homolog 1

NaN, sodium channel subunit $\beta 2$

NSC, neural stem cells

OP, oligodendrocyte progenitors

PAMPs, pathogen associated molecular patterns

PNET, pancreatic neuroendocrine tumor

PRRs, pattern recognition receptors

PDGF, platelet-derived growth factor

PDGFR, platelet-derived growth factor receptor

PET, positron emission tomography

PyV, polyomavirus

REC, retinal endothelial cells

REF52, rat embryonic fibroblasts

ROCK, rho-associated protein kinase

RPTPβ, receptor protein tyrosine phosphatase β/ζ

RNAi, ribonucleic acid interference

RT-PCR, reverse-transcriptase polymerase chain reaction

qRT-PCR, quantitative real-time polymerase chain reaction

SCC, squamous cell carcinoma

scFv, single chain variable fragment

SELEX, systematic evolution of ligands by exponential enrichment

SF, scatter factor

siRNA, small inducing ribonucleic acid

SIP, small immunoprotein

SMART, simultaneous multiple aptamers and RGD targeting

SMOC1, SPARC-related modular calcium-binding protein 1

SOCS, suppressor of cytokine signaling

SPARC, secreted protein acidic cysteine-rich

SVZ, subventricular zone

TA, tenascin-C assembly domain

TEC, tumor-derived endothelial cells

TGFβ1, transforming growth factor beta 1

Th cell, T helper cell

TIMP, tissue inhibitor of metalloproteinase

TLR4, toll-like receptor 4

TNIII, fibronectin type III-like repeats in tenascin-C

TNC, tenascin-C

VEGF, vascular endothelial growth factor

VN, vitronectin

Wt, wild type

www.ingramcontent.com/pod-product-compliance
Lightning Source LLC
Chambersburg PA
CBHW061326220326
41599CB00026B/5059